The Fitness Groove

How to Never Stop, Never Give Up and Finally Stay Fit Forever!

Dr. Scott Lewis

BREAKTHROUGH ENTERPRISES
LAS VEGAS, NEVADA

To my grandfather,

Milton Lyle

Cover Design: Dunn+ Associates
Interior Design: Marin Bookworks
Illustrations: Grizzly Graffix

Lewis, Scott, 1963-
    The fitness groove: how to never stop, never
give up and finally stay fit forever!/Scott Lewis. — 1st   ed.
    p.cm.
        LCCN: 99-94608
        ISBN: 0-9666224-1-3

        1. Physical fitness—Psychological aspects. 2.
Motivation (Psychology) I. Title
    GV481.2.L49 1999   613.7'01'9
                                              QBI99-454

Manufactured in the United States of America
Breakthrough Enterprises
2810 W. Charleston Blvd., #H-84
Las Vegas, Nevada 89102
(888) 427-5847

Acknowledgments

The author wishes to acknowledge Joe "Mr. Fire" Vitale, Cindi Anderson, Dan Kennedy, John Runnette, Elaine Vernon, Charlotte Spielberger, Sharon Goldinger at PeopleSpeak, Robin Cantor-Cooke, John Kremer, Dan Poynter, Denise Kovac, Dottie Walters, Victoria Rhine at Grizzly Graffix, Melvin Powers, and John Hendrickson, Esq., for their support and guidance.

Special thanks are also extended to friends and family: Dr. Revina Lewis, Norman Lewis, Mary Lyle, Joe and Lori LoCicero, Betty Gliner, Joel and Rhonda Lyle, Dr. Sheri Frazin, Tom and Janyne Oblonsky, Lance Burton, Peter and Coral Reveen, Liz Tucker, Greg Auston, James and Paulina Brandon, Carol Chehade, Evan Klingsberg, Claudette Moore, Jim and Amy Ream, and Mark Yuzuik.

Contents

Introduction

Have you ever begun an exercise program, only to abandon it three weeks later? Do you constantly start and stop participating in fitness routines because you get too busy for them or lose your motivation? Do you want to lose weight and improve your health but find you are unable to do so? If any of these situations sound familiar, or if you have always wanted to incorporate a fitness program into your life, *The Fitness Groove* can help you.

I have worked with more than a thousand people for the past eleven years and found that the key to obtaining results from any fitness program is follow-through. So much emphasis is placed on starting a program that once you've begun, you often neglect what you need to do to stay consistent and get results. As a wise man once said about his cigarette habit, "Stopping smoking is easy—I've quit hundreds of times."

It's your ability to stay consistent and follow through with your fitness program—what I call being in the

Fitness Groove—that will lead to success. Although the weeks and months of continuing your program will not be as dramatic as the day you begin, it's the discipline of follow-through, not the drama of beginning, that will change your life. You may have ambitious fitness goals and start out strong, but if you don't have staying power, you will never achieve the results you want from your program.

And isn't this true in other areas of life? Consider romance. Many relationships start off strong but soon disintegrate because all the couples had was the excitement of novelty. The couples that stay together are the ones who find novelty and excitement in the ordinary, everyday routines that life is made of. And the same holds true for business. The most successful businesspeople don't achieve their fortunes overnight. Starting a business is one feat; growing it into a success is another. Day by day, successful people do what is necessary to build their businesses. Initiating action is important, but it takes one only so far. In romance, business, and fitness, it's following through that counts.

This book will help you find and stay in the Fitness Groove by providing the tools you need to successfully start and continue your program. Follow-through is the most important factor in a successful fitness program—it's what keeps you in the Fitness Groove and achieving results.

I've designed this process so that you're doing and not just thinking. So I'm not going to talk a lot about theory because even if you learn everything there is to know about human physiology, you still might not be able to follow through with your fitness program. After all, if book learning were all that was required, there wouldn't be any fat physicians.

Once you're able to get into the Fitness Groove and stay with your program, you will be on your way to achieving the results you want. Of course, your program needs to be one that deserves the energy you'll be putting into it, so throughout this book you'll find lots of tips on how to ensure that your program stays worth your while.

So put on some shorts, lace up your athletic shoes, and grab a towel—this book is about taking action. If you've always wanted to start a fitness program, or if once upon a time you started one but didn't follow through, this book is for you.

Let me show you how to get in the Fitness Groove and start experiencing the results you've always dreamed of!

Let's Get Started

The first step toward successful follow-through is starting out right. You can't follow something through until you've started it, and by starting your program right, you will maximize your chances of staying in the Fitness Groove.

Before you start, choose the type of exercise you want to do. Don't worry about finding the perfect exercise; many kinds of exercises in various combinations or on their own will allow you to achieve your goals. Of course, certain types of exercises are better suited than others for achieving particular goals. If you want to lose weight, improve your cardiovascular health, or both, you will probably want to focus on aerobic activity. "Aerobic" means "with oxygen," and aerobic activities are those that get your blood pumping and elevate your heart and respiratory rates over a sustained period. Activities such as running, cycling, using a rowing machine, or climbing virtual flights of stairs on a stepping machine can all be forms of aerobic exercise.

On the other hand, if your goal is to add muscle mass to your body, you will probably focus on strength training (lifting weights). Strength training is typically considered an anaerobic activity because even though you're breathing regularly, you are not raising your heart or respiratory rate for a sustained period nor are you using large amounts of oxygen while you exercise.

Is All Strength Training Anaerobic?

Some experts make an exception for circuit training, a strength-training regimen where you complete a series of weight-lifting tasks over a sustained period with a minimal amount of rest between sets. Completing the circuit can take half an hour or more. Some people would consider circuit training an aerobic exercise, while purists would still call it anaerobic. I'd probably call it subaerobic.

It's also important to remember that you don't need to focus on just one type of activity. If walking on a treadmill becomes tiresome for you, try a stair-stepper. If you get bored exercising alone, take an aerobics class. You're more likely to follow through if you enjoy what you're doing, and with all the options available nowadays, there's no excuse for getting stuck in a workout rut. In fact, it's beneficial to alter your routine because your body will respond better when you surprise it with a change in activity. For example, try incorporating strength training into your program if you've been doing only aerobic activity or incorporating aerobics if you've only been lifting weights. I'll explain more about the benefits of cross-training later on.

Once you've chosen the type of exercise(s) you want to do, commit to following through. The best way I've found to accomplish this is to make your commitment official. You don't have to buy yourself an engagement ring, but you do have to set a date to start your program—no backing out, no rain dates, no excuses. Most people need to feel that they have officially started their programs to remain consistent. Otherwise, it's too easy to miss a workout or two and say "I'll start for real after my sister's wedding" or "There are only six days left in the month; I'll start on the first of next month."

These aren't commitments, they're noncommitments. They don't work. If you start your program in this way, it will be easy to abandon it because you won't feel as if you ever really started it.

Setting a Date

You must set a specific date to begin your program. Tell your friends when you'll be starting your program. Make the day meaningful by telling yourself This is my official date and I'm not going to change it. Make the date so significant you'll feel bad if you break it and have to choose another, less meaningful one. This is why many people make New Year's resolutions: It's a new year, an official opportunity to start fresh. We get this opportunity only once every 365 days, and we are all eager to redeem ourselves, even if our resolve lasts for only a few weeks. We know this is a once-a-year offer, and if we break our promises, we have to wait another year before we start fresh again.

Look at your calendar, determine a day that has some special meaning for you (even if it's solely because it's the day you've designated), and commit to starting your program on that day. It can be today, it can be tomorrow, it can be a week from tomorrow, or it can be even a month from tomorrow. Just pick a day on which you know you will be able to start. And if you pick a day that is significant to you for other reasons, that's even better. Maybe you'll start on your birthday or an anniversary or your child's birthday—whatever you like.

Take a moment now and select a start date. When you've picked one, write it down in the space below:

I will start my exercise program on

_____

Good! You just took an important step toward establishing a successful fitness program. Now I want you to write this date on small slips of paper and place them around your house. Be sure to make enough, especially if you live in a big place. I want your start date to be with you wherever you are. Put one on the bathroom mirror, type it into your electronic organizer, circle it on your calendar, and trace it in your child's sandbox. Remind your friends and family of your plans and become emotionally invested in this day.

As I said before, if you can't start right away, choose a future date on which you can start. If you're reading this on the Wednesday before Thanksgiving, give yourself a break—start your program on Monday. Don't structure your program on shaky ground. I'd much rather have you start when you're likely to succeed.

Again, remember to let people know about your commitment. Tell the world! Don't make the mistake of thinking you can start your program quietly so that if you don't follow through with it, you won't have lost anything and can start again later. Decide whom you want to tell, pick up the phone, get in your car, go online and send out some e-mail—just get the word out. By letting others know about your commitment, you will establish a group of people you can rely on to provide support and

---

Debbie

Debbie was a waitress and forty-two-year-old mother of three who had struggled to control her weight for most of her life. Throughout the years she had started many fitness

(continued)

programs but was never able to stick with any of them long enough to get results.

The turning point for Debbie came one day before her forty-third birthday when she was able to clearly visualize herself at a lighter weight and felt a wonderful sense of pride and self-confidence that she hadn't experienced in years.

With a renewed sense of purpose, Debbie made a decision that night that she would start her program on her birthday. She didn't want to be overweight another year, and the significance of her forty-third birthday offered her the perfect opportunity to start her program. On the next day, her birthday, Debbie started her program. Within four months, she had accomplished her goal of losing twenty-eight pounds and was back at her ideal weight. Debbie had found her Fitness Groove and hasn't looked back since.

encouragement and keep you on track when your resolve starts to falter. You are the main player in this game—there's no question of that—but even the greatest players love to hear the cheering section.

The Secret to Success:

Identifying Your Compelling Reason

You've set a date and committed it to writing. Your house is covered with Post-it® notes and other reminders of the day on which you'll officially begin your program. You've told your friends about it as well all the members of your family and every neighbor within a three-block radius. You're all ready to go—and then, all of a sudden, the "what ifs" start creeping in.

What if I can't stay motivated and follow through? What if I start and then stop two weeks later, the same way I did the last time I decided to get in shape? What if I don't have the discipline I need? What if I'm the fattest person in my aerobics class? What happens when I use the machines at the gym and everyone looks at me? What if everyone else is twenty years younger than I am?

I've heard these "what ifs" for years. Over and over again I've heard about programs that people couldn't stick with and about people not having enough time, losing motivation, growing discouraged, and abandoning their programs. And for years I've been asking myself why people give up on their programs—why they can't stay in the groove, why they lose their momentum, why they lose heart and quit.

A while back, I finally found the answer, and it's based upon an important principle: If you want to accomplish something, *give yourself a good reason for doing it.* For instance, have you ever known someone who wanted to quit smoking and tried his or her hardest for a day or a week or even a month but just couldn't kick the habit? I've known folks like this, people who have smoked two or three packs of cigarettes a day for years, who have tried to quit numerous times using a variety of methods—nicotine gum, patches, computer programs, you name it—but who have never been successful. Then, one day, all of a sudden, they quit "cold turkey" and never put a cigarette in their mouths again. Why are they suddenly able to quit? How do they do it?

Compelling Reason

Experts have found that the most important factor in changing any behavior is having a compelling reason for doing so. Perhaps a woman learns she is pregnant and cares enough about her baby's health—and her own—to flush her Marlboros down the toilet. Maybe a forty-five-year-old man who has been smoking half his life watches his father die slowly of lung cancer and suddenly finds that lighting a cigarette seems like one small, glowing step toward a long and painful illness. Something clicks in the brain, an effect is connected to a cause, and a person who felt powerless to change one day is transformed the next.

Of course, not everyone reacts this way. Some smokers hack and cough their way through hundreds of cartons of tar and nicotine. For them, the thought of imminent death isn't frightening enough to make them quit. For others, vanity accomplishes what fear cannot. I heard about a woman who finally quit smoking when she read in *Reader's Digest* that smoking could accelerate the wrinkling around her eyes.

My family has its own story as well. My grandmother Mary, who smoked for twenty years and developed a bad cough and other health problems, quit on the day I was born because my mother said she wouldn't let her near me as long as she continued to smoke.

We all have our reasons for doing what we do, and that's exactly the point: When you identify *your* reasons*

---

*Your emotionally appealing reason may actually be several different reasons, and that's okay. For simplicity, I will refer to the motivation that drives you to reach your fitness goals as "your reason" not "your reason or reasons."

for doing what you do, you clarify your purpose and see your life in terms of choices you make, rather than events that happen to you. When you identify your reason for wanting to be fit and healthy, you clarify your purpose for creating an exercise program and establish a way to stay committed to it. This commitment is at the heart of being in the Fitness Groove.

Consider this example of the importance of having a good reason to be fit. Have you ever wanted to lose weight for an upcoming wedding or high school reunion? I have two questions: First, did you succeed in losing the weight you wanted to, or at least a good portion of it? You probably did. Why? Because from the moment you opened the invitation, you focused on all the benefits you were going to receive by losing weight and looking your best. You weren't thinking about how deprived you were going to feel when you skipped dessert, ate butterless bread, and denied yourself Southern fried chicken and fries for six weeks. No, you visualized how terrific you were going to look in your wedding gown or tuxedo or Italian sport coat or little black dress, and you imagined how satisfying it would feel to hear everyone tell you how wonderful you looked. To put these appealing thoughts into action, you might have started taking the stairs instead of the elevator, parking in a space a bit farther away from the mall, or walking around the neighborhood for fifteen minutes each night.

Second, once the honeymoon was over or the reunion ended and the balloons and streamers came down and you were back at work the following Monday, did you maintain your new, lower weight and continue looking your best? Chances are you didn't. Once the big event was over, you probably stopped focusing on all the benefits you had reaped from becoming fit and you reverted to your old routines—buttering your bread, ordering dessert, and eating great big pieces of greasy, golden-brown, extra crispy chicken. You began taking the elevator up the two flights you used to climb and eyeing enviously the handicapped parking place in front of the department store. Once you lost your compelling reason, it was easy to put off doing what you needed to do to stay at your goal.

If I were to ask you if losing weight was still important to you, you would probably say yes—especially if you were overweight. But without a compelling reason driving you to do what you need to do, without a mental picture of the benefits you'll receive by being fit, typically it's much more difficult to accomplish your goal.

Your Own Reason

You undoubtedly are aware of the dangers of being overweight and sedentary—increased chances for heart disease, diabetes, and numerous other ailments. Yet while important, these facts may not motivate you to engage in regular exercise.

But what about the thought of how confident and terrific you'll feel when you slide into that pair of jeans you've been avoiding for the last two years? Would that get your attention? Maybe that's the key to your motivational strongbox: the pleasure of having your body look more attractive to others and feel more solid and vibrant to you.

You may have other reasons besides wanting to increase your physical attractiveness. Maybe you want to improve your general health and be able to run up a flight of stairs without getting winded, awaken with vitality, and have more energy throughout the day.

The key is to find out what truly motivates you. The importance of this principle cannot be emphasized enough. Whatever your reason for wanting to be fit and healthy, it's up to you to determine what it is. Once you have figured that out, you're on your way.

If you already know what motivates you, great. The SEARCH method you will learn in chapter 3 will help you strengthen your resolve. And if you cannot articulate right now what motivates you, don't worry. We'll deal with that in the next chapter. You have to establish your own personal motivation. It all comes back to you. You need to look inside yourself and identify your compelling reason—the vision that will feed the fire inside you. Once you've found your fire, you must commit to stoking it every moment of every hour of every day. And once you've got it burning brightly, that fire will keep you motivated and on track for days and months and even years.

But before you can stoke your fire, you must get it started. That's what we'll be doing next.

Ben

The process of quitting smoking is an example of how powerful having a strong, emotionally appealing reason can be. Ben was a businessman who had smoked two to three packs a day for the past twenty-five years. For many years, he had tried almost everything ever marketed to stop smoking, including aversion therapy, but he was unable to quit.

Ben was finally able to stop smoking in a single session by focusing on how his life would be different as a nonsmoker. He realized that he'd have time to get more done at work and be able to spend more time with his family. He visualized the smiles on his wife's and son's faces as he came home an hour earlier every day. This realization alone was so powerful and compelling to Ben that he was able to stop smoking instantly and successfully remain a nonsmoker.

The SEARCH Technique:

Changing Your Approach to Fitness Forever

For years the SEARCH technique has been extremely effective in helping people reach their fitness goals. SEARCH stands for Seeking Emotionally Appealing Reasons to Change (and Create) Habits. By using this technique, you will be able to identify your true source of motivation—your emotionally appealing reason for wanting to be fit—and this will help you follow through with your program and stay in the Fitness Groove.

Some motivational techniques can help you get started on a program by creating a sense of excitement; others can give you a temporary boost that gets you into the gym every now and then after the initial thrill wears off. Wearing a headset and listening to music to keep you climbing a stair-stepper is great for getting you through that portion of your workout, and watching television while you're on a stationary bicycle can distract you from the repetitive nature of the activity. But while these techniques are effective for keeping you focused on a specific activity for a specific amount of time, they can't do what the SEARCH technique does: reveal to you the underlying visceral and emotional motivation that will propel you through your program and on to success.

The SEARCH technique is unique in several ways. First, while it helps you actively search for your emotionally appealing reason, it also helps you relax. It is much easier to focus on your emotionally appealing reason when you are relaxed. Second, the technique encourages you to use your imagination. It is designed to trigger thoughts that help you define what is truly important to you. Third, within the SEARCH technique is a special process called SEARCHLINK, which helps you establish a personal signal you can use any time you wish to be reminded of your compelling reason. Last, with every use, the SEARCH technique will reinforce your special reason, helping you to stay highly motivated.

SEARCHLINK

A fascinating example of the proverbial mind-body connection is how emotional states can be triggered by certain physical signals. These physical cues can involve sight, sound, touch, taste, or smell. For example, you may

(continued)

hear the same song that was playing when you ended a relationship four years ago and suddenly feel sad. Or you may smell a certain perfume or cologne and instantly long to be with a favorite person you associate with that particular fragrance. Or perhaps as a child you fell through a lake covered with ice and forever feel tentative walking over iced surfaces.

By using the SEARCHLINK process, you can establish a special physical signal that you can link to the enthusiasm you feel as you visualize your strong emotionally appealing reason for participating in your program. By establishing this link, you can re-experience this strong motivating reason whenever you use your signal. I've found cues involving touch to be the most convenient and have suggested in the scripts (see appendix I) closing one of your fists, touching your forehead with your fingertips, or touching your thumb and index fingers together as good signals you can use. Of course, you don't have to use these suggestions and can develop your own signal.

To use the SEARCHLINK process most effectively, decide on the signal that you will be using and when you first listen to the SEARCH tapes (described below), perform this signal when instructed to. Ideally, you should perform your signal at the very moment you're in your most excited state—visualizing all the wonderful benefits you'll be obtaining from your fitness program. The stronger the emotional state you're in when you perform your signal, the more powerful link you'll establish.

Of course, I recommend listening to the SEARCH tapes numerous times, so with each listening you'll be able

(continued)

to reinforce your signal. Also, after the first time you listen to the SEARCH tapes, you do not need to perform your signal precisely when you're instructed to on the tape. Any time you feel a height of excitement about all your compelling benefits, perform your signal.

By establishing a link between your compelling reason and your signal, you'll have the ability to remind yourself of these exciting benefits whenever you choose. If you decide not to establish a signal, you can still benefit from the SEARCH technique simply by thinking about your compelling reason often.

Making the SEARCH Tapes

To use the SEARCH technique most effectively, you'll need to get a tape recorder and make an audiotape of yourself reading the scripts that start on page 115 in appendix I. There are two scripts: one for SEARCH Technique I: How to Find and Lock In Your Motivation and one for SEARCH Technique II: Designing and Achieving Your Ideal Body. The scripts are similar but not identical. The first one will help you relax your body and evoke a serene feeling while you search for and "lock in" your emotionally appealing reason. The second will aid your search by helping you relax your body and focus on how you would like to change it. By recording yourself reading these scripts and then listening to them, you will guide yourself through the process and accomplish your goal. The SEARCH technique works best when you can put yourself into a receptive listening mode—free to use your imagination while you listen to what you have recorded.

Your Voice

I strongly suggest that you make the effort to record the scripts yourself. The SEARCH technique is an important tool that will be useful to you, and you should use both scripts. Also, making the recordings will be tangible proof that you are willing to take the steps to make your program a success. If you don't like the way your voice sounds on tape, or if you feel strange listening to your own voice giving you instructions, have someone else record the scripts for you. (Special recordings of the scripts are available. See the order form at the end of the book for more information.)

The Soundtrack

I also suggest that you play a relaxing soundtrack in the background when you record the scripts. Some people find nature sounds comforting and like to hear ocean waves, trickling streams, or chirping crickets while they are engaged in the SEARCH process. If this appeals to you, go to a well-stocked music store and look through its collection of environmental recordings. You should find a large variety to choose from.

Other people prefer to have music in the background, and this can work, too, as long as it doesn't distract you from the script. Whether you prefer music or environmental sounds, it is important to use a sound-track that relaxes you. Don't use *Tales from the Vienna Woods* if you're allergic to pine trees. Similarly, if classical music annoys you, you might prefer an easy listening version of "Hotel California." Any background music will work as long as it has a relaxing effect on you.

Practice

Read the scripts a few times before you record them. This will familiarize you with the material and enable you to read it without faltering and with more expression, emphasizing words and phrases that you find particularly effective. Don't worry that reading the scripts in advance will somehow diminish their novelty or "spoil the surprise." After all, the plan is for you to use these tapes over and over again. After the first listening, the surprise is gone.

The usefulness of the tapes lies not in their novelty but in their repetition, so their effectiveness will not be lost if you read the scripts before you use them. In fact, by reading the scripts before you record them, you will create better recordings and gain more benefits. You may find that after recording the scripts and listening to the tapes a few times, you're not satisfied with the way they sound. If this happens, record them again, changing your inflection or the speed with which you read or the loudness of your voice. Adjust your reading in any way necessary to get an effective recording.

The Tape

Go ahead and get a tape recorder and a blank audio-tape. Each script is about twenty minutes long. A sixty-minute tape will enable you to record one script per side and have about ten minutes of blank tape left over. When you've listened to one script, you can fast-forward and cue up the other side. If you use a ninety-minute tape, you may be able to record both scripts on one side, depending on how fast you read. But you will have to rewind the entire tape when you have finished listening to the second script in order to cue up the first one again (unless you're very ambitious and record both scripts on both sides of the tape).

No matter what length audiotape you use, make the recording. If you don't own a tape recorder, buy one (you can get a hand-held model for about twenty dollars) or borrow one from a friend. Do whatever it takes to get these tapes recorded. If you have not yet embarked on a fitness program, fine—record the scripts. If you are in the midst of a fitness program, that's also fine—record the scripts. The SEARCH technique is that important—regardless of where you are in your quest for fitness. Using this technique is at the heart of staying in the Fitness Groove.

When the tape is made, take it out of your recorder and punch out the little plastic tab on the cassette shell. If you don't punch out the tab, you may inadvertently erase the tape if your finger touches the record button.

Removing the little plastic tab makes it impossible to erase or record over your recording. If you later want to rerecord your scripts, place a small piece of cellophane tape over the opening where the tab used to be, and you will be able to record again.

When you have finished recording your scripts and are happy with the way they sound, read chapter 4. Chapter 4 contains additional information you need to use the tapes properly, so don't start using the SEARCH technique until you read it.

See you there!

Judy

Judy was one of the first patients of mine who used the SEARCH technique. Judy was a delightful woman employed as an advertising executive. She had heard about the work I was doing and came to me for assistance in getting back on her fitness program.

For two years, Judy had steadily gained thirty-five pounds—a result of abandoning a three-times-a-week aerobics class she had previously much enjoyed. Judy had become so busy at work that it seemed impossible for her to find the time to get to the gym. Week after week, she'd promise herself that first thing Monday morning she'd start back on her program. But on Monday morning, instead of being at the gym in her aerobics class, Judy would be behind her desk and working on the company's latest campaign.

(continued)

What Judy was able to discover by using the SEARCH technique was how important it was for her to feel attractive. Although she was successful at work and was happily married, Judy was unhappy with her body's appearance and sad that she had let herself get out of shape. While using the SEARCH technique, Judy remembered in great detail how pretty she used to look and how wonderful she used to feel hearing all the compliments she'd receive whenever she wore her favorite red dress—a dress she hadn't been able to fit into for over a year.

The day following our session, Judy started back at her gym with a new focus and the exciting vision she obtained during the SEARCH technique of wearing that red dress again and receiving compliments on how terrific she looked. Work was still hectic, but with a new awareness of how important it was for her to be thinner, Judy was now taking the time to work out. Within five months, she had returned to her ideal body weight and was able to proudly wear that special red dress to her family reunion.

Judy is one of thousands of people who have derived tremendous benefits from the application of the simple yet powerful SEARCH technique.

Using the SEARCH Tapes

Congratulations! You've recorded the scripts for the SEARCH technique. The tapes that you have created are powerful tools you can use any time you wish to sharpen your focus and boost your motivation. Remember that the key to getting motivated and staying in the Fitness Groove is to have an emotionally appealing reason for doing what you're doing.

The most effective way to use these tapes is to listen to them in a place where you can close your eyes and remain undisturbed. You should never listen to the tapes when you're driving a car or doing anything else that requires your full attention because the tapes encourage you to close your eyes and will tend to make you drowsy.

Don't worry if you're not able to visualize everything that the scripts ask you to. Some people are able to picture everything in great detail, while others get more general images. You don't have to visualize every word for the process to be effective. The more you listen to these tapes, the clearer your emotionally appealing reason will become. Many people find that as they listen over and over again, they are able to relax more fully and focus more clearly on their reasons.

If you're interrupted while you're listening, stop the tape, attend to whatever you need to, and when you're ready, resume your listening. Just because you're relaxed doesn't mean that you're incapable of directing your attention back to the external world.

Picturing Your Compelling Reason

When you use the tapes, you will establish your emotionally appealing reason for starting and sustaining your program. Once you've figured out what's inspiring you, you must maintain a constant awareness of what you are working toward. When you identify your compelling reason for wanting to be fit and healthy, picture it in your mind and keep it there, at the front of your thoughts, all the time. (And remember to use your signal.)

If you want to get back into those slim-cut jeans, picture how good you used to look in them (or if they were always too small, picture how good you'd like to look in them) and how great you used to (or will) feel in them.

If you want to be healthy so you can watch your children grow up, picture their glowing faces and feel how precious they are to you. When you do this each time you exercise, your workouts will be more meaningful. You will know that every time you get on that stair-stepper, hop on your bicycle, or participate in any other physical activity, you'll be getting closer and closer to your goal. And you won't lose your focus and get caught up again in the routines of daily life. If you do find yourself slipping back into old patterns and losing your motivation, listen to the SEARCH tapes and strengthen your resolve anew.

Using the SEARCH technique to identify your emotionally appealing reason for getting fit can also help you control your eating habits. When you are following through and exercising regularly, you will begin to see and feel results. Maybe you'll run up a flight of stairs without gasping for the first time in ten years, and when you reach the landing, maybe your belly won't be jiggling as much as it used to either.

You will experience these results organically—you'll feel them and know them in your body, in your bones. So when those perfect cannolis come rolling by on the pastry cart, they may look good, but not as good as you do in your jeans. You may be tempted to order dessert, but you will also realize that fitting into your old jeans will make you feel a lot better than eating a dessert ever could. By keeping a picture of your goal in the front of your mind, you will keep yourself motivated, and that means being able to change unhealthy eating patterns that you were never able to change before.

Once again, your goal is to focus constantly and unflinchingly on all the benefits you will obtain by following through with your program. It may seem difficult at first, especially when you have not yet begun to see results. But by following through with your program and using the SEARCH technique, you'll be able to stay in your groove and achieve the results you're after.

Unconscious Eating

The SEARCH technique can help you change your eating habits. Many people slip into an "unconscious" mode of eating whenever they dine.

When you're constantly aware of the goal(s) you're working toward (e.g., fitting into that special outfit or looking great on the beach), you have the power to make the best food choices possible. This isn't to say that you can never again have a slice of apple pie—you can. It's just that you're now able to put the (caloric) cost-benefit ratio into perspective.

We all indulge from time to time, and it's perfectly okay to do so. You'll find, though, if you have constant awareness of what your exciting vision is for yourself, you'll be able to make more objective decisions about what to eat rather than eating just for the sake of eating, which often means eating more than you should.

Flexible Scheduling:

The Key to Being Consistent

So far, we've looked at three steps you should take to get started on your program and follow through with it:

1. Set an official start date.

2. Determine your emotionally appealing reason for starting and sustaining a fitness program.

3. Keep this reason at the front of your mind.

The purpose of this book is to show you how to start with your program and follow it through, and the cornerstone of successful follow-through is being consistent. If you are exercising moderately—even if this means only two to three times a week, every week—you are going to see results faster than people who ambitiously start out exercising five times a week, only to find they cannot maintain that schedule and sabotage themselves by starting and stopping all the time. We all know the moral of the story of the tortoise and the hare: Slow and steady wins the race. Life doesn't always arrange itself around you and your goals, no matter how sincere your commitment to them may be.

That brings me to the next point: when you design your exercise regimen, it's important to keep in mind something I call flexible scheduling. It means exactly what it sounds like: building flexibility into your workout schedule. Too many people set themselves up for failure by setting unrealistic goals. They say, "I'm going to work out ninety minutes a day, every day, no matter what." And when they miss a day because they have the flu or they are away on business and stuck in meetings until midnight, they say, "That's it. I've ruined my program. I'll have to start over when I can do it right. Maybe after the holidays." Does this sound like anybody you know? Does it sound like you?

This is a common, black-or-white, all-or-nothing attitude that many people exhibit when they embark on a new course in their lives. The inner voice of this attitude sounds like this: "Either I'm going to do my program flawlessly or I'm not going to do it at all. And since I can't do it perfectly right now, I'm going to stop and start over again when I *can* do it perfectly. Sure, I've worked out five times a week for the past three weeks, but I missed yesterday's workout so I've broken my perfect schedule. I'll wait until next Monday when I can start all over again."

Or how about this excuse: "I had a jelly doughnut at the staff meeting this morning and I can't go to the gym tonight to work it off. If I can't do it right, I'm not going to do it at all. I'll start over again next week when I can be good."

Don't get caught in this trap! It is inevitable that one day you will schedule an exercise session and be unable to follow through and complete it. Sooner or later, someone will bring jelly doughnuts to the staff meeting. To try to be perfect is an unrealistic goal as well as an unreasonable one, and you will sabotage your finest efforts if you think perfection is possible.

If you are flexible when you schedule your exercise sessions, you will be able to follow through with your program and stay in your groove for a long time—even forever. Instead of telling yourself that you've got to work out every night of the workweek or swearing that you'll be at the gym on Mondays, Wednesdays, and Fridays, do this instead: promise yourself that you will exercise two or three times a week. That way, if you plan to exercise but for some reason cannot, you will still be on schedule if you work out the next day or the day after that. (To help you keep track of your workout schedule and the progress you're making, use the Personal Success

Logbook, starting on page 142, which is designed to encourage flexible scheduling.)

Exercising two or three times a week is an attainable goal; expecting to always exercise on the same days or at the same time is not. Life is too unpredictable for you to stick to a rigid workout schedule. When you structure your exercise schedule, build some flexibility into it. That way, though you may have to bend your rules, you don't have to break them, and your commitment will remain strong.

My Own Experience

Until I discovered the SEARCH technique and flexible scheduling, I was never able to be consistent with any exercise program. I was one of those "all or nothing" people. I had to do my program perfectly; otherwise, I wouldn't do it at all. After I hit a personal "rock bottom" in 1993, severely overstressed and thirty-six pounds overweight, I was able to finally turn myself around by discovering and applying this powerful technique.

Results

Let's talk about results and the important role they play in keeping you in the Fitness Groove.

One of the main reasons that people get frustrated and abandon their programs is that they don't see results soon enough. A person who has been exercising regularly for three weeks might wake up one morning, step on the scale, find that he has lost only two pounds, and think, Who am I kidding? This isn't worth it. I'm not seeing *any* results. Why should I keep knocking myself out, running to the gym (or three miles around the neighborhood) three times a week if it isn't going to make a difference? (Of course, the results are there. He just doesn't know where to look for them.)

Does this scenario sound familiar? If so, take heart: there are ways to handle these feelings of frustration. One of the best ways is to be realistic about your goals. Yes, looking terrific in your swimsuit is a strong, emotionally appealing reason for starting a fitness program. But if you've just started working out again after eight or ten years of spending evenings on the couch in front of the television, it's going to take some time for you to reach your goal. I'm not saying you should stop picturing yourself looking terrific on the beach—quite the opposite! It's important that you see yourself as you wish to be and keep an image of your emotionally appealing reason in the front of your mind. Remember, even if your goal seems way out of reach right now, that's fine. To lose weight, improve your level of fitness, or sculpt your physique, you have to start somewhere.

It's important to measure your results in small, recognizable increments. Rather than view success as the achievement of your ultimate goal, you must instead identify your starting point and measure your results in intervals that you recognize as significant.

People often forget how they looked before they started their programs and miss an excellent opportunity to reinforce the fact that they are indeed making progress. Your progress may manifest itself in subtle ways: your face may start to appear less full, your arms may grow more toned, your stomach might bulge less above your waistband. If you don't create a basis for comparison, you might miss these changes and deprive yourself of the opportunity to reinforce your resolve.

If your goal is to have more energy and improve your health, take a moment to jot down a few notes in the space below about your present level of health. Do you get winded climbing the flight of stairs to your friend's apartment? If so, write this down. If you can walk only a block or two before you need to stop and rest, make a note of this as well. These notes will help you identify your starting point.

What's Your Present Level of Health?

Here's a space for you to jot down your observations. Refer to this later as you assess your progress.

_____

_____

_____

_____

_____

_____

_____

As you continue with your exercise program, refer to these notes to remind yourself of how well you are doing. And remember to be realistic: you might not be able to bound to the top of the Eiffel Tower—at least not right away—but you will be able to visit your friend without showing up on the doorstep gasping for breath. And that's significant progress.

If your goal is to build muscle and improve your physique, snap a few pictures of each area you are trying to build. Besides being a source of motivation as you monitor your progress, these photographs will become great "before" shots that can be used to motivate others when you have achieved your goals.

It's important for you to realize that by participating in a regular exercise program you are changing your life: You are changing both the way your body looks and the way it works. You are making the right move! Remember that, just like good things, worthwhile results come in small packages. When you consistently follow through with your program, your results will be consistent as well. Remember to evaluate your results at small intervals and celebrate each small success because the accumulation of these small successes will lead you to your goal. Stay consistent! Stay in the groove!

Finally, if your goal is to drop pounds and lose fat, don't become discouraged, abandon your exercise program, and embark on one of these gimmick diets that promise fabulous results in only thirty days. Any weight you lose in one month will soon pile back on. These gimmicks don't work, and in the next chapter, I'll show you why. I'll also show you the best ways to measure your results. You may be surprised to learn that a scale is not the best place to measure your progress.

Measuring
Your Results:
Where to Look

By now, you know that your emotionally appealing reason provides a strong motivation for you to stay in the
Fitness Groove. You also know that another powerful
motivation comes from seeing results. What you may not
know is where to look for results and what to look for.
The results you seek will differ depending on whether
your fitness goal is to lose weight, improve your overall
health and well-being, or build muscle—or even a com-
bination of all three. Here is a description of what to look
for in each of these categories.

If Your Goal Is to Lose Weight

The most important rule is to stay off the scale. That's right—stay off the scale. This may sound confusing because in the last chapter I discussed how important it is to pay attention to the results you're achieving. The important distinction is to make sure that you are measuring your results *accurately*. That innocent-looking bathroom scale will often mislead you. To measure your progress solely by its readings is a big mistake, especially if you're trying to lose weight.

Different Kinds of Weight

Why isn't a scale a reliable indicator of how much weight you're losing? Because you may say you want to lose weight, but what you really want to do is lose fat— and muscle weighs more than fat. If your program involves strength training, you are going to be building muscle. Even if your program consists solely of taking aerobic workout classes several times a week, you are still building muscle (albeit in smaller amounts).

Adding muscle weight is highly beneficial to your fitness program, but you may feel as if you are failing if you step on the scale after your first month of exercise and find that you have lost only four pounds. After all, when you've been working hard, sweating off what feels like quarts of water, and pushing your body to what feels like its limits, you don't want to find out that you weigh only four pounds less than when you started, even if the reason is that you've lost five pounds of fat and gained a pound of muscle.

On the other hand, losing twenty-five pounds in one month may seem like a tremendous victory. But rapid weight loss is rarely sustained. In most cases, people gain the weight back—and often more than they lost—within a short period of time. This is precisely why I urge you not to step on the scale if your primary goal is to lose weight (or rather, fat).

Scale readings are often deceptive and not a reliable indicator of your results. I would much rather have you lose five pounds of fat in one month and gain a pound of muscle than lose twenty-five pounds of water, muscle, and some fat; have the scale give you a false sense of accomplishment; and watch you put all the weight back on over the next few months.

Why is muscle so important? Because the amount of muscle your body has is one of the factors that determine your metabolism, the rate at which your body burns calories. Muscle tissue burns a tremendous amount of calories. So it follows that increasing your amount of muscle creates a greater need for calories, which is beneficial for weight loss. When you try one of those gimmick diets and lose twenty-five pounds in one month, only some of the weight you have lost is fat—the rest is muscle and water. Although you are proud of what the scale says and feel as if you have made progress, you have actually lowered your need for calories. This is why once you end the diet, it's so easy to gain back the weight you lost.

Your Measurements

So how do you measure your progress if you can't rely on the scale? That's easy: take your body measurements before you start your program. The only tool you need is a tape measure. (The fabric kind sold in sewing stores works well. The metal kind sold in hardware stores usually isn't flexible enough and can be awkward to use.)

To measure your waist, wrap the tape measure around your waist (or where you remember your waist used to be) and across your navel. (See illustration 1.) Hold the tape closed in front with one hand, and write down the measurement with the other. (Record your measurements in your logbook so you can monitor your progress.) To measure your hips, wrap the tape around the part of your body below your waist where you are the widest. (See illustration 2.) Write down that measurement, too.

Measure your waist and hips every few weeks as you continue with your program, write down your measurements, and monitor your progress. You might not notice steep weight drops if you step on the scale, but you will notice that your clothes fit better. This is because you are losing inches in your waist and hips. Whether you are adding muscle through strength training or toning muscle with aerobic exercise, you are still increasing your body's percentage of muscle. Muscle is more compact than fat, so when you are involved in a fitness program and are building muscle and losing fat, you are tightening your physique. Just picture a bodybuilder and you'll know what I mean.

Body Fat

Another good way to assess your progress is to measure your body fat. The process by which this is accomplished is based upon the principle that your body weight consists of two elements: fat and lean body mass (bones, muscle, organs—everything in your body except fat). By figuring out how much fat you are carrying, you can judge how well you are doing.

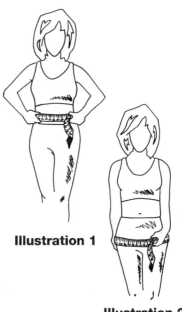

Illustration 1

Illustration 2

One of the most reliable ways of measuring body fat is through underwater weighing. This involves sitting on a scale, expelling all the air from your lungs, and being submerged in a specially constructed water tank. Since fat weighs less and floats more readily than lean body mass, people with high amounts of body fat are more buoyant than those with less fat. Using this principle, underwater weighing measures a body's percentage of fat based upon that body's floatability when suspended in the tank. While this method is reliable, it can be inconvenient if you don't have access to a weighing tank. Additionally, some people feel uncomfortable expelling air from their lungs and then being submerged in the tank.

Fortunately, there are other ways to measure body fat. Various electronic and other high-tech devices have been developed that claim to be highly accurate at measuring body fat. Before you decide to purchase one of these, I recommend that you make sure it carries a money-back guarantee, because while some devices are quite good and warrant the expense, others function best only as places to store batteries or as modernistic living room décor.

Skinfold Calipers

One inexpensive, convenient, and reliable way to measure body fat is to use skinfold calipers. These are widely available and recommended by many fitness experts because they are accurate to within a few percentage points and easy to use.

The trick to using skinfold calipers is to pay careful attention to what you are doing: measuring the amount of fat that has accumulated under your skin at specific sites on your body. The amount of fat under your skin (called subcutaneous fat) is a fairly accurate indicator of your total amount of body fat. To get an accurate reading, at each site, with your thumb and forefinger, pinch together the skin and fatty tissue that lies directly beneath the skin (see illustrations 3a and 3b), being careful to lift them away from the muscle underneath. Do this directly on your skin, not through clothing. With a little practice, you will recognize the squishy feel of fat between your fingers and be able to know when you are effectively lifting it away from the firmer, more substantive muscle. (Picture yourself eating a piece of chicken and think of how different the meat feels from the fat that sometimes comes with it.)

Once you are confident that you have properly pinched together the skin and fatty tissue, substitute the calipers for your fingers (see illustration 3c) and take a reading. (Most calipers come with instructions on precisely where to place them—for instance, half an inch from where your fingers are pinching, a quarter of an inch from your fingers, and so on.) If you've pinched and placed the calipers properly, you will get a fairly accurate reading of the body fat you are carrying at that site. For even greater accuracy, you can repeat the measurement three times and use the average when computing your body fat percentage.

When you use calipers to calculate your body fat, specific places on the body should be tested. Opinions vary on the number of sites that should be measured and what these sites should be. Illustrations on pages 50–52 show some of the commonly recommended sites. You can use these as a general reference, but do use the sites specified in the instructions that come with your calipers. A chart will also usually be included with the calipers so you can determine your body fat percentage based upon the readings you obtain.

It is important that you be consistent when you use calipers and measure the same sites every time you take readings. A good way to make sure you are checking the

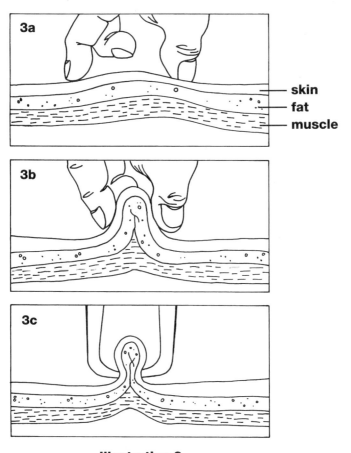

Illustration 3

same places every time is to use a tape measure to mark each measuring site. For instance, if you are using your left triceps muscle (located at the back of your arm) as a measuring site, use the top of your left shoulder as a landmark to locate the pinching spot on your triceps. Hold one end of the tape measure at the top of your shoulder and measure down about three to four and a half inches, whatever length is appropriate for your arm, to find the right spot for your triceps pinch. Every time you use the calipers on your left triceps, make sure you are pinching the same spot by using the tape measure.

Also, don't be shy about asking someone to help you take your measurements. Certain sites may be hard to reach by yourself, and if you try to measure them alone, you are likely to take inaccurate readings. To keep measurements consistent, be sure that the person you recruit is available to help you on an ongoing basis or has made accurate notes that can be followed by someone else.

Ideal Body Fat Percentages

You're probably wondering what ideal body fat percentages should be. Most experts recommend that men's bodies be about 15 percent fat and women's bodies be about 22 percent fat (women naturally have more fat than men). It is well documented that we risk many health problems if we carry extra body fat. Many American men and women have body fat percentages that far exceed healthy limits and put them at greater risk

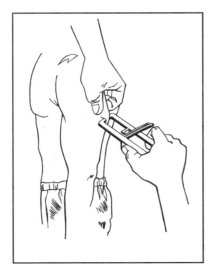

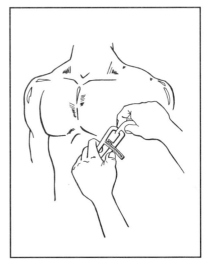

Illustration 4   **Illustration 5**

for developing high blood pressure, heart disease, adult-onset diabetes, and even certain cancers.

The good news is that you can decrease your body fat by exercising regularly. As you lose fat and gain muscle, your body will be affected in two ways. First, since you are losing fat, your body fat percentage will decrease. Second, because you are gaining muscle, your lean body mass will increase, and since more muscle means more calories are burned, this can lower your body fat, too. So if your body doesn't look or feel the way you would like it to, don't fret over your fat. Instead, follow through with your program, stay in the groove, and take body fat measurements regularly, about every two weeks. The results you see will be a true indication of your progress and far more reliable than the readings you could get from a scale.

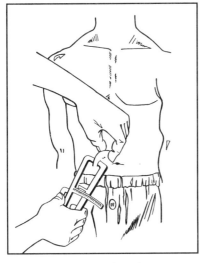
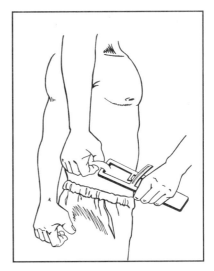

Illustration 6   **Illustration 7**

If Your Goal Is to Improve Your Health and Fitness

Taking hip and waist measurements and calculating body fat percentages will provide most people with a good indication of the progress they are making in their health and fitness programs, as well as in their efforts to lose fat. Decreasing abdominal fat has been proven to decrease the chances of heart disease, especially in men. However, if you are already slender, I do not recommend that you take frequent hip and waist measurements. Rather, you should probably be putting your energy into building muscle to ensure you won't become too thin.

Just as body fat measurements are useful for determining how much extra fat you're carrying around, these measurements are also useful for determining if you have

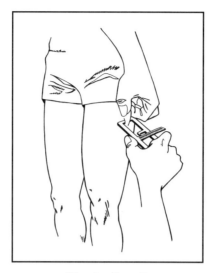

Illustration 8

too little fat on your body. I know it is said you can never be too rich or too thin, but I take exception. You *can* be too thin.

Of course, if you're an athlete in peak condition, you may be able to have a much lower percentage of body fat than is recommended and suffer no ill effects. But if you're not preparing to try out for the U.S. Olympic gymnastics team, it's probably better to keep your body's fat percentage near the recommended amount. Women may stop menstruating if their body fat percentage falls too low, and both men and women can become vulnerable to various ailments if they allow themselves to get too thin.

Your Resting Heart Rate

Another way to gauge the success of your fitness program is to determine your resting heart rate when you first start your program and keep track of it as you progress. Resting heart rate refers to the number of times your heart beats every minute when your body is at rest—that is, when you are relatively still. This is also referred to as your resting pulse rate.

It is important to understand that resting heart rates vary from person to person due to heredity, fitness level, and other factors. Typically, the more fit you are, the lower your resting heart rate will be. When you exercise regularly, your heart becomes more efficient and can deliver more blood and oxygen with each beat so it doesn't have to beat as frequently as does the less efficient heart of an out-of-shape person. Athletes sometimes have resting heart rates as low as thirty to forty beats per minute, while out-of-shape folks may have resting heat rates of over ninety beats per minute.

Again, there is good news: you can lower your resting heart rate by following through with your exercise program and improving your level of fitness. Monitoring your resting heart rate and watching it decrease can be exciting proof that you are indeed improving your fitness level.

If you see your resting heart rate *increase* significantly—that is, a difference of ten beats or more per minute—you may be overtraining or overexerting yourself. Become familiar with the symptoms of over-training so you can tell if you're overdoing your workout. You may feel unusually tired or have difficulty sleeping (or both); you may experience nausea or diarrhea or frequent colds; you may feel disoriented, have difficulty concentrating, or become depressed or unusually irritable.

Pay attention to your body. Don't force yourself to exercise for the sake of sticking to a schedule you devised when you were feeling relaxed and well rested. (Remember flexible scheduling!)

Many cases of overtraining can be treated by resting for a day or two (in other words, for twenty-four to forty-eight hours, don't exercise). If you think you may be over-training, it's far better to nip the problem in the bud and take a day or two of rest. If you don't rest and instead continue to push yourself, you may have to take off weeks or even months to fully recuperate.

How to Measure Your Heart Rate

To accurately measure your resting heart rate, you need to know how to take your pulse. One of two sites is commonly used—the radial artery, located on the underside of each wrist near the base of the thumb (see illustration 9), and the carotid arteries, which run along both sides of the neck (these are the vessels you see throbbing when someone gets very angry) (see illustration 10). To measure your resting heart rate, choose one of these two sites. Rest your index and middle fingers gently over the

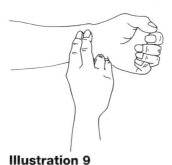

Illustration 9

artery you are monitoring. You should be able to feel gentle pulsations. You will count them to determine your resting heart rate.

Don't use your thumb because it has its own pulse that you may end up counting in addition to the artery's. When using your index and middle fingers, don't press too hard, as deep pressure may alter your reading. It's a good idea to measure your resting heart rate as soon as you awaken in the morning while you are still in bed and feeling calm. If you wait and measure it after you have arisen, made breakfast for your children, and downed two cups of coffee, you will probably not get a true at-rest reading.

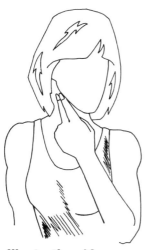

Illustration 10

Once you have found your pulse and are applying the proper amount of pressure, count the pulsations for a full minute. Write down the count in your logbook and continue to measure your resting heart rate regularly as you follow through with your program. You may even measure it daily if you wish to.

Your Recovery Heart Rate

Another way to measure your fitness level is by monitoring your recovery heart rate. To do this, take your pulse immediately after completing your exercise routine, wait one minute, and take your pulse again. The more fit you are, the quicker your heart rate will drop toward its resting rate and the quicker you will have "recovered." Since exercise conditions vary, taking recovery measurements is not as accurate an indicator as taking resting heart rate measurements, but you can frequently see improvements when you compare your recovery times at the start of your program to those you achieve after your program is in full swing.

If Your Goal Is to Gain Muscle

All the measurement techniques mentioned so far are valuable sources of information even if gaining muscle is your primary (or exclusive) goal. Since your body fat percentage will decrease as your lean mass percentage increases, you will be able to monitor your muscle gains by using body fat measurements. If you were to rely solely on the bathroom scale, you would have no way of determining whether the weight you gained was muscle or fat.

Muscle Mass

When measuring your muscle mass or girth, it is best to use a flexible cloth tape measure. First, find the spot where the muscle is the widest and wrap the tape measure completely around that area. Then, take your reading. Remember to use a joint or other body part as a landmark to be sure you are measuring the same part of the muscle each time. You can also measure different areas of the same muscle to get a more detailed picture of your progress. For instance, if you want to measure your thigh, you may either measure the widest part of your thigh, as suggested above, or measure the thigh in three different places—the part that's closest to your knee, the part that's closest to your hip, and the part that's the widest. Once you've taken your measurements, don't forget to write them down. (An area for recording your measurements is included on each of the strength training progress sheets in the logbook.)

Strength

Finally, you can also gauge your progress by monitoring how much weight you're able to lift. As you progress with your strength training program, you'll be able to lift more and more weight. Even if you're lifting in order to tone rather than build your muscles, the amount of weight you're able to lift will still probably increase because it will become too easy for you to lift the amount of weight you started with. As you may have guessed, when you start a strength training session, it's a good idea to review how much weight you lifted last time. You can do this easily by looking at your logbook, where you will be keeping a record of how much weight you've been lifting.

Don't feel you have to lift more weight than you did at your last session or even the same amount. Don't push yourself to the point of overtraining—or worse, injury. If the weight feels too heavy, lighten it. Many people sprinkle some lighter workout days into their strength training schedules because not every day needs to be intense in order for a program to work.

Eat Enough Calories

Before turning to how hard and how often you should be working out, there's something even more important to mention: nutrition—eating food and eating *enough* food. You have to eat enough calories. This may sound obvious if your goal is to build muscle, but it might not have occurred to you if your goal is to lose weight. The fact is, even if your goal is to lose weight, you must eat a sufficient number of calories in order for this to happen successfully.

What do I mean by *successfully?* You already know that all weight loss is not the same. Many people think losing weight means merely that: you get on the scale and you weigh less this week than you did last week—hooray, you're losing weight! A common attitude is that it doesn't matter what you're losing as long as your body is carrying fewer pounds around than it used to. This just isn't true; what you're losing *does* matter. To repeat, when you lose weight, you are not necessarily losing fat; you may be losing water and muscle as well. And when you don't consume enough calories, you are certain to lose muscle tissue as a result of your body's adaptations to the severe caloric restriction you are placing it under.

How Much Is Enough?

What is the minimum number of calories you should be consuming? Most experts agree that you need at least 1200 calories a day if you are a woman and 1500 calories a day if you are a man. People who go on ultralow-calorie diets think that they're doing themselves a favor, but since these diets lead to a loss of muscle tissue, they've done themselves no favor at all. Losing muscle for the sake of losing weight will cause you trouble in the long run.

You already know that the more muscle mass you have the greater your body's need for calories. Why would you want to do anything that would cause you to lose muscle? You will constantly struggle to keep your weight down if you lose muscle because you lose valuable calorie-burning "engines." Even if your fitness program consists entirely of strength training, you will sabotage your program and lose some of the muscle you are working so hard to build if you do not supply your body with sufficient calories.

Additionally, with these so-called prison diets, your metabolism will slow down as your body attempts to conserve energy. It doesn't know that you're skipping breakfast and eating only carrot sticks and rice cakes because you want to. It thinks that someone has locked you in a dungeon and is trying to starve you to death. Since your body has no idea how long you will be in this predicament, this adaptation makes sense.

Yes, people lose weight on ultralow-calorie diets. But because some of the pounds they are losing are pounds of muscle, the moment they go off their diets and resume their old eating habits, they gain the weight back. Even if they change their habits and eat smaller portions, they still tend to gain the weight back because their bodies have lower caloric needs. This is what is known as yo-yo dieting, or weight cycling, and you don't want it to happen to you. Not only is it counterproductive, it is also dangerous. After all, if your body keeps losing muscle tissue, it can eventually lose muscle from your vital organs, including your heart.

Finally, when you don't consume enough calories, your energy level drops, and it's very hard to follow through with a program when you feel you don't have the energy to change into your workout clothes, much less spend twenty minutes on the stair-stepper. Yes, you've lost weight, but you've also lost your energy, your drive, your ability to motivate yourself. If you want to burn fat and have the energy to follow through with your program, you have to eat enough calories. When you starve yourself, your biggest loss is your spirit, and that doesn't show up on the scale.

The Importance of Water

I'd also like to discuss the importance of drinking water. Undoubtedly, you've heard that you should drink at least eight cups of water a day. Water is one of our body's most vital nutrients, and we need to ensure we drink enough because we lose water in our waste products as well as when we're breathing and perspiring—which is to say, all the time.

Anyone who is involved in physical activity, spends a lot of time in the heat, or is involved in any other situation where water loss is accelerated has an even higher need for replenishment. Unfortunately, many people participating in fitness programs are unaware of this or do not place enough importance on drinking sufficient quantities of water.

A surprising fact is that you can be in a state of dehydration and not even know it. This occurs much more frequently than you'd think because by the time we feel thirsty, we are already slightly dehydrated. We are not able to physiologically sense dehydration beforehand (and this sensitivity often decreases with age), so we must rely on our own discipline to drink enough water.

What happens when you become dehydrated? First of all, your blood becomes thicker, does not flow as easily, and becomes less efficient in delivering oxygen to your muscles. Can this affect your performance? Of course it can! Without an adequate nutrient supply, your muscles are unable to perform as well and they become much more quickly fatigued. How are you going to stay on that elliptical machine long enough to burn fat when your muscles tire quickly? Additionally, your performance can suffer if you experience any of a number of other symptoms of dehydration, for example, muscle cramps, headaches, and disorientation.

When dehydration becomes severe, the very dangerous conditions of heat exhaustion and heat stroke can occur. Without sufficient water, your body's ability to regulate its temperature becomes impaired, and with heat exhaustion and heat stroke, your body's temperature rises dramatically. Under normal conditions, you lose water through perspiration, which dissipates heat that builds up within your body. Naturally, when you're involved in physical activity, you perspire more. When you're significantly dehydrated, the water in your body is used mostly to supply oxygen and nutrients to your muscles, and is used less for sweating. When your body loses the ability to efficiently dissipate heat by perspiring, your body temperature rises. If it continues to rise, you may find yourself in a life-threatening situation.

Obviously, the point of this discussion is to make sure you're drinking enough water. Don't wait until you're thirsty to drink water, especially if you're involved in an exercise program. It is okay to drink water while you are exercising. (But you might want to slow down or pause for a moment so you don't spill it all over yourself.) It's a good idea to drink at least one-half cup for every fifteen to twenty minutes you are involved in exercise. It's also important to have a cup before you start your activity and especially important to have at least a cup after you've finished. You should probably have even more when you are done with your workout if you feel as though you have been sweating a lot.

It is also important to make sure that you're drinking water throughout the day. Many people find this easiest to do when water is conveniently available. Of course, it's easy to accomplish this by carrying a bottle of water wherever you go. Take it to work, keep it in your car, carry it with you when you walk your Doberman. Not only will you function better, but you'll also have more energy as well. Please realize, though, that it is actually possible to drink too much water, and this can create health problems as well. Because you're involved in an exercise program, drinking nine to twelve eight-ounce cups a day is reasonable. Of course, everybody is different. Some people may require a little more, others a little less.

One other bit of information—not all beverages are the same. You may think that the water content in colas and alcoholic drinks will help keep you from getting dehydrated. Actually, the opposite is true. Both alcohol and carbonated beverages have a dehydrating effect on your body, so watch your intake of those rum and Coke drinks!

Keep this quick course in nutrition in mind. The benefits of increased performance and better health that you'll obtain by consuming enough calories and drinking enough water will enable you to more easily stay in the groove, follow through with your program, and achieve the results you're after.

The FIT Principle

Now that you've decided never to starve yourself again on one of those gimmick diets and have promised to make sure you eat right and drink enough water, let's move on to the FIT principle. (FIT stands for frequency, intensity, and time.) Once you understand how to use this principle to your advantage, you will be able to accelerate your results and improve your follow-through.

Since the variables of frequency, intensity, and time for aerobic exercise differ from those for strength training, each will be covered separately.

Aerobic Exercise and the FIT Principle: Frequency

Let's start with the *F* part of the FIT principle: frequency. Of course, the more frequently you exercise, the more benefits you will enjoy. If you are able to work out four or five times a week, you will see results faster than you will if you are able to work out only once or twice a week. That's logical. But as I've been saying all along, it is still better to work out twice a week regularly than to plan on working out five times a week and not do it.

If you are able to exercise frequently, make sure that you allow yourself at least one day off every week. Your body needs a day to rest, and working out every day for the next fifteen days is not a good idea, especially if you're very out of shape or just starting your program. Also, as we get older, our bodies need more rest. Whatever your situation is, you may feel the need to rest a day between sessions, and that's fine.

Aerobic Exercise and the FIT Principle: Intensity

The *I* in FIT refers to intensity. Most people have a huge misconception about this concept. They think that in order to get the maximum benefit from an exercise session, they have to be gasping for air, with their lungs burning and faces contorted with strain. No wonder so many people think exercising isn't any fun!

It all comes down to physiology. If you want your body to burn fat, it must have enough oxygen to do the job. If you're exerting yourself so much that you're gasping for air, your lungs aren't getting enough oxygen and your body can't burn fat efficiently. If you keep this up too long, the fat-burning process will virtually shut down. You have to slow down and allow your body to get the oxygen it needs to do what it wants to do: burn fat.

Your Training Zone

Many experts recommend that you exercise in something called "the training zone" if you want to achieve optimal results from your fitness program. In simple terms, the training zone is a range of heart rates within which your heart should be beating as you exercise. The traditional method of determining your training zone has been to calculate your maximum heart rate—that is, the fastest rate your heart can beat—and then to define a range of rates not exceeding the maximum within which your heart should beat as you exercise.

You can calculate your maximum heart rate by subtracting your age from 220. For example, let's say you are thirty-three years old. Two hundred twenty minus thirty-three equals 187; therefore, your maximum heart rate would be 187 beats per minute.

To locate your training zone, you need to calculate a percentage of your maximum heart rate. Experts vary in their recommendations, but most agree that your training zone should be approximately 60–80 percent of your maximum heart rate. As paper and pencil (or a calculator) will show you, 60 percent of 187 beats per minute is 112 beats per minute, and 80 percent of 187 beats per minute is 150 beats per minute. Therefore, with a maximum heart rate of 187 beats per minute, your training zone would be a heart rate of between 112 and 150 beats per minute.

Now that you know how to calculate your training zone, don't be compulsive about it. Recent research shows that the 220-minus-age formula may not be consistently accurate for a significant portion of the population because using age as the sole determinant of a person's maximum heart rate is problematic. Why? Because not all sixty-year-olds have the same fitness profile, and neither do all forty-eight-year-olds.

According to the age formula, your maximum heart rate goes down as your age goes up, thus a sixty-year-old man would have a maximum heart rate of 160, while a forty-eight-year-old man's would be 172. But a sixty-year-old who runs five miles three times a week is likely to be in better shape than a forty-eight-year-old couch potato and would probably have a higher maximum heart rate than his sedentary (albeit more youthful) counterpart.

Also, research now shows that genetics play a role in determining your maximum heart rate. Some people have naturally faster- or slower-than-average heart rates, and their maximum heart rates would not be accurately calculated using the 220-minus-age formula. As you can see, it is not so simple to accurately determine your maximum heart rate, and it is therefore equally difficult to determine your training zone. That is, if you base your *personal* training zone on the *average* for your age, you may calculate a range that is either too low or too intense for your body's maximum benefit.

Since the 220-minus-age formula is still frequently cited in books and charts as a way to determine your maximum heart rate and training zone, it is important that you be aware of its limitations. If you are gasping for breath and feeling lightheaded but you still haven't reached what your calculations describe as your training zone, listen to your body and slow down. Don't trust a mathematical formula when your living, breathing (and gasping) body is telling you something else. A formula cannot take into consideration your fitness level—which changes, after all—or your genetic makeup. Your body is the more reliable information source.

The Talk Test

An easier and more effective way of determining a suitable intensity level is to use the talk test. It's very simple: while you are exercising, you should be able to carry on a conversation with the person on the treadmill next to you—using short phrases, that is. So if the man on your right asks where you got your cross-training shoes and all you're able to say is "The mall," that's fine. You should exercise at a rate where you're panting a bit but still able to convey coherent snippets of information. If you can't even grunt out two syllables, then you're exercising too intensely for optimal fat burning to occur. On the other hand, if the man to your right asks where you got your shoes and you say, "Oh, I got them at the mall at a health food store that happens to have a shoe department in the back. You know, about seven doors down from where Saks Fifth Avenue just opened up," then you probably haven't reached your ideal intensity level.

Please note that I said *ideal* intensity level. If you're just starting your program and aren't comfortable panting even a little bit, don't worry. Start exercising at a level that is comfortable for you. You can always increase the intensity to your ideal level later when you are more fit. Remember that you don't have to exercise at hyperkinetic levels in order to become healthy and fit. If you're working out to the point of exhaustion, your body isn't able to burn fat efficiently, you run the risk of overtraining, and you are sabotaging yourself.

By the Numbers

Another way to gauge intensity is to develop a numerical system to estimate how hard you are exercising. For example, you might decide to use a system ranging from zero to twelve, where zero would represent the amount of effort you would put into watching television on the couch, while a rating of twelve would represent the most extreme, gasping-for-air, couldn't-go-any-harder-if-my-life-depended-on-it level of exertion. Under this system, a rating of six might represent a moderate level of exertion, while higher numbers such as eight, nine, and ten might represent levels where you're breathing rapidly (but still within the guidelines of the talk test), your pulse rate has increased, and you're perspiring.

This sort of numerical system has been written up in fitness literature as the "rating of perceived exertion," or RPE, and typically uses a scale that ranges from zero to twenty. Some experts use a scale ranging from zero to ten, but what matters is not how many numbers are on your scale but whether the scale makes sense to you. Decide on a scale that you can use and then consistently record your rating in your logbook. Using this system, you will be able to monitor your progress as you start exercising more and more intensely.

Remember, too, that the same principles apply here as to the talk test—you don't want to be at the extreme end of your scale if your goal is to burn fat. The training zone—60–80 percent of your maximum heart rate—is where most experts recommend you work out if you want to burn fat. It's a lot easier to follow through and stay in the groove when you know you can achieve results without feeling as if you're about to collapse.

Aerobic Exercise and the FIT Principle: Time

The *T* in FIT refers to time. Obviously, the more time you spend exercising each session, the more fat you will burn. This is because at the beginning of your workout, your body is burning carbohydrates (sugars) more efficiently than it is burning fats. Sugars are easy to burn and a good source of quick energy, while fats take longer to start burning and are an excellent source of sustained energy. As you continue exercising, your body will burn fats more efficiently, especially when you've been exercising for about thirty minutes; for most people, that's when significant fat burning starts to take place.

The longer you can continue working out at your ideal intensity level, the better the results you will achieve in the long run. If you start a session too intensely, you won't last long. And if you don't last long enough, you might stop exercising before you reach the magic thirty-minute mark. If you're new to exercise, you may want to start slowly so you will be able to exercise longer and burn fat more efficiently. If you can devote a little more time to each of your workouts, you will get better results in less time as you follow through with your program.

Strength Training and the FIT Principle: Frequency

Because strength training—working out to build muscle and increase strength—tends to be anaerobic, the frequency guidelines for this kind of program are different from those for an aerobic program.

For instance, with aerobic programs—those geared primarily to burn fat and improve cardiovascular health—the more frequently you exercise, the more progress you will make as long as you're not overtraining.

But if you are engaged in or embarking upon a strength training program, it's probably a good idea for you to rest at least one day between sessions. This is because strength training sessions place a lot of stress on your muscles and you need a day to repair and increase the muscle mass you are working on. If you don't give your body adequate time to recover and repair itself, you will diminish your results. Now, some serious bodybuilders spend six days a week at the gym and seem to suffer no ill effects. For the most part, though, they are using advanced techniques and doing so many different exercises, they can emphasize different muscle groups on different days and avoid overtraining.

Many people who are new to strength training will begin with a three-days-a-week schedule, working out, for example, on Mondays, Wednesdays, and Fridays or on Tuesdays, Thursdays, and Saturdays. This is a sensible way to start a program, and it enables your body to recover enough to follow through. Of course, you should always be flexible with your scheduling and remember that even if you must miss a few days, your results won't suffer much. Just make sure that missed days don't grow into missed weeks or you will need greater assistance from the SEARCH technique.

Another way to schedule a strength training program is to split your routines and work different muscle groups on different days. An example of this would be to work the muscles of your upper body on Mondays and

Thursdays and the muscles of your lower body on Tuesdays and Fridays. (Wednesdays and weekends are skipped to give your body a chance to rest.) Although you are working out two days in a row in the Monday-Tuesday and Thursday-Friday sequences, your body still enjoys the effects of a rest period because you're working different muscle groups on consecutive days. Unless you are training for high-level competition, working out three to four times a week is enough in a strength training regimen.

Repetitions and Sets

Before discussing intensity, it's important that you understand the term as it applies to strength training; and to do this, it's important to know about repetitions and sets. If you have trained before, you are familiar with these terms. If you are new to the process, a short explanation will be helpful.

Repetition refers to the number of times you lift a weight and return it to its starting position. Say, for example, you were building your biceps muscle with a hand-held dumbbell and you were standing. You would start the exercise holding the dumbbell at your side. You would then proceed to lift the dumbbell up toward your shoulder, contracting the biceps. Once you had contracted the muscle as much as you wanted to, you would then lower the weight to a relaxed position at your side.

The up-and-down motion would be counted as a single repetition, and you would then go through the same up-and-down motion for your second repetition. (You may hear somebody using the technical terms for these movements: the upward, lifting motion for this particular muscle group is referred to as the positive or concentric phase of the cycle, and the downward, lowering motion is referred to as the negative or eccentric phase.)

That's one repetition. A group of repetitions constitutes a set. So if you did eight repetitions for your biceps muscle, rested a few minutes, and did another eight repetitions, you would have performed two sets.

Strength Training and the FIT Principle: Intensity

Now let's talk about intensity. An important component of intensity is the amount of weight that you lift with each exercise. When you start a fitness program and for the first few weeks afterward, you should be lifting weights that you can manage easily. Don't feel you have to do fifteen different exercises; you can start out effectively by doing only a few. Don't worry about how hard you can push yourself. Instead, use this time to familiarize yourself with the equipment and get your form right. Do a set of ten to fifteen easy repetitions for a muscle group, and then move on to the next group. One set of repetitions for each muscle group is enough when you're starting out. As you progress, you can add more sets to your program and increase the amount of weight you're lifting.

There are many opinions about how to manage a strength training program. How many repetitions should you do? How many sets? When you are determining what level of intensity to strive for, many factors play important roles. I have reviewed much of the research on this issue and found that most studies' recommendations on the best intensity levels for strength training fall within a common range.

Many recommend two or three sets for each muscle group consisting of six to ten repetitions per set. Of course, a serious weightlifter often will have a different program. To determine how much weight you should be lifting, many experts suggest that you choose a weight that you can lift a maximum of ten times per set. When it starts getting easy to do ten repetitions and you feel that you would like to do more, you should start increasing the amount of weight you are lifting, usually in small increments.

Because there are so many variables among the factors that constitute a good strength training program, you need to find out what works best for you. You will notice that I have not included a list of specific strength training exercises you should be doing. This is because there are hundreds of different ones and everybody (as well as every body) responds differently to exercise. The perfect program for one person may not be effective for you. Many excellent resources are available—hundreds of books, audio programs, and video programs have been created on this topic—as well as knowledgeable trainers you can consult at your local gym. Finding out what works best for you and following through with your strength training program will bear palpable results.

Strength Training and the FIT Principle: Time

In any strength training program, the amount of time you spend will be determined by the number of different exercises you wish to do and how many repetitions and sets you perform. Also, the time you spend training will be influenced by the amount of time you take to rest between sets and exercises. Most experts recommend that you take at least a thirty-second break between sets. You may want to wait even longer. There's no rule saying you can't wait longer if you want to, and you may want to use the opportunity to drink some water.

Finally, don't forget to breathe! It's not unusual for people starting a strength training program to actually forget to breathe, gritting their teeth and holding their breath as they lift and lower the weights. If you don't keep inhaling and exhaling regularly, you can increase your blood pressure, place stress on your heart, get dizzy, and even pass out. Although strength training is considered anaerobic, you still need to breathe so your body gets oxygen.

Whether your fitness program consists mostly of aerobic exercise or of strength training, you will enhance it tremendously by paying attention to the frequency and intensity with which you exercise and the time you devote to it. You can experience even better results by combining aerobic exercise and strength training, which you'll read more about in the next chapter.

Cross-Training:

Dramatically Improving Your Results

Cross-training means doing different forms of exercise. Runners may cross-train by cycling. Swimmers may cross-train by lifting weights to build up their upper bodies. Cross-training is good because it breaks up the monotony of doing the same activity all the time. It also helps decrease the likelihood of injury because atheletes are not using the same muscles in the same motions over and over again. Cross-training has received a lot of attention in recent years because of its increased use in competitive athletics.

You can cross-train by doing different aerobic activities. If you consistently work out on a stair-stepper, you can cross-train by jogging. You can also cross-train by mixing your aerobic exercise with strength training—a great way to enhance the effects of an aerobic workout program. When you integrate aerobic exercise, used primarily for its fat burning and cardiovascular benefits, with strength training, used primarily for building and strengthening your muscles, you can accelerate your results dramatically.

Integrating Strength Training and Aerobic Exercise

Since you now understand the relationship between muscle mass and burning calories, you can appreciate the benefits of building muscle. If your program is primarily aerobic—in other words, you use a treadmill, stair-climber, stationary bicycle, and so on—you can improve your results, especially those associated with fat burning, faster by adding strength training to your program.

Usually, aerobic exercise will only slightly increase muscle mass. If you really want to build muscle, you must train for strength. This does not mean you have to spend two hours a day, five days a week at the gym. Effective strength training can be accomplished in as few as twenty-five minutes a day, two or three days a week.

If you own home equipment, it is important that you know how to properly use it. Be sure to read the instructions that come with the equipment *before* you start using it. Also, there are many excellent books and videos that will teach you proper technique. If you're going to be using the equipment at your local gym, talk to the people there who have been trained to assist you. Most gyms have people on staff who can show you how to use the equipment, design a program specifically for you, and even supervise your first few workouts to make sure that you are doing the exercises correctly. You can even hire a personal trainer to provide you with a little extra motivation and assistance. Even if your technique is already good, small bits of advice here and there can make a big difference in your results. With strength training, there is always a potential for injury, and it's worth spending some time, effort, and even extra money to learn to use the equipment properly.

A common misconception is that strength training is beneficial only for young people. This is completely untrue. Numerous studies have shown that strength training is beneficial for all age groups—even for people in their nineties! In fact, strength training has been shown to be particularly effective in combating some medical problems commonly afflicting people over sixty. As people age, their muscles atrophy if they don't use them, and some people can lose up to 40 percent of their muscle mass. When this happens, they may lose the ability to lift even light objects, to walk up stairs, even to walk at all. It's important to do some form of strength training as we age to lessen the chances that we'll find ourselves unable to do these basic tasks.

Another hazard of aging, especially in women, is osteoporosis, a condition in which the bones lose density and become brittle, weakening the skeleton and making the bones more likely to break. Areas that are most likely to be affected are the wrists, the spinal column, and the top of the femur (the hip). Osteoporosis is a leading cause of hip fractures, many of which can be fatal because of complications. Osteoporosis can also lead to compression fractures of the vertebrae, resulting in decreased height. Strength training and weight-bearing exercise put stress on bones and cause them to respond by becoming denser; it also builds up muscles. So by exercising for strength and building muscle, people suffering from osteoporosis, as well as those not so afflicted, can add stability to their bodies' frames. Strength training can also help maintain coordination in people of mature years and make it less likely that they will fall. Of course, you should speak with your physician before embarking on a strength training regimen, especially if you are sixty years old or more, as there are some medical conditions for which strength training would *not* be beneficial.

Another common misconception about strength training is that women who practice it will bulk up their muscles and look like men. This is also untrue. I know what you're thinking: what about those professional female bodybuilders on television whose muscle definition is just as extreme as that of their male counterparts? The difference is that those women have spent hours upon hours, days upon days, weeks upon weeks, and often years upon years training with the express purpose of creating this effect. (It is also not unusual for female bodybuilders to ingest steroids—hormones that promote muscle growth.) For most women, adding some muscle mass decreases flabbiness, provides their bodies with a tighter look, and accentuates their natural curves by supporting them with a solid muscle base. Remember, if you feel you are building too much muscle, you can always cut back on your strength training regimen and train just enough to stay toned.

For both women and men, adding muscle is one of the best ways to lose fat. Your body burns fat to maintain its muscle mass, and by adding muscle you raise your metabolism and the rate at which your fat is burned. This is why you may have heard that if you increase your muscle mass, you can burn fat more effectively even while you sleep. Because your body is metabolizing the calories you ingest twenty-four hours a day, increasing your muscle mass will cause you to burn more fat both when you are at rest and when you are active.

Finally, strengthening your muscles plays an important role in helping you prevent lower back pain, an ailment that afflicts over thirty million people every year. Lower back pain often occurs when muscles that have gradually weakened are suddenly forced into a movement that they're no longer strong enough to support. You bend down quickly to pick up your twenty-seven-pound toddler, or you're at a wedding and dancing up a storm for the first time in years, and suddenly a searing pain knives across your back that makes you stop dead in your tracks and gasp in surprise. And the pain doesn't stop when you do; it remains for hours or days or even longer. Sometimes you will see a chiropractor for relief. I've treated hundreds of cases like this. This kind of lower back pain can be prevented by maintaining strength in the lower back and abdominal muscles, which provide support to the central region of your body. And there's nothing like strength training to get those muscles in shape.

Integrating Aerobic Exercise with Strength Training

Because strength training does not sustain your heart rate as aerobic activity does, adding aerobic exercise to your strength training program will improve your cardio-vascular system in ways that strength training alone cannot. Even if you incorporate aerobic exercise only a few times a week, your strength training routine will be more balanced and produce more health and fitness benefits.

Also, strength training alone will not provide you with the fat-burning effect of aerobic exercise. For instance, if your abdominal muscles are a bit flabby, you can do hundreds of crunch exercises, but you won't get that washboard stomach until you do something about the fat that's there. To lose the fat most efficiently, you need to do aerobic exercise.

Keep in mind that if you're a serious bodybuilder, incorporating aerobic activity will typically not improve your performance. To gain the maximum amount of muscle, it's usually best to stick with a strength training program. If you're not planning to compete in body-building competitions, however, you can reap tremendous benefits by incorporating aerobic exercise into your strength training program.

Warming Up
and Stretching:

Benefits You May Never Have Realized

Warming up and stretching before you exercise can significantly affect your ability to follow through with your program and stay in the groove. Many people neglect to include these simple processes because they are either unaware of their importance or not sure how to do them. In this chapter, you'll learn why warming up and stretching are so important and how you can easily incorporate them into your program.

Perhaps the most obvious benefit of warming up and stretching is that these activities dramatically lower the chance that you will injure yourself during your workout. A body whose muscles have grown pliable through a thorough warm-up and stretching routine is a body ready to perform. If you jump right into your activity without warming up, using tight muscles that haven't been stretched, you're more susceptible to strains and sprains. When you suffer such an injury, you disrupt your workout schedule and often end up on the sidelines for weeks (or sometimes even months), losing the results you've worked so hard to achieve. It's hard to follow through with your program when you're injured.

In addition to preventing injuries, warming up and stretching can help improve your performance. When you warm-up, you increase the blood flow to your muscles, and more oxygen and nutrients are delivered. Also, because the temperature of your muscles increases (hence the term "warming up"), your muscles can use oxygen more easily, which improves your performance. When you stretch, you increase the flexibility and range of motion of your muscles so you're able to work your muscles more thoroughly and efficiently, which means you can burn more calories during aerobic activity and build more muscle during strength training.

Warming up before exercising is important because of what may happen to your heart if you don't—especially if you haven't yet reached a high level of fitness. If you jump right into an intense activity, your heart can become stressed and react in unpredictable ways. Obviously, this defeats the purpose of exercising to improve your health. You need to warm-up, stretch out your muscles, and start slowly so your body has time to catch up and adapt to your increased activity level.

By now, you should be convinced that warming up and stretching should be a part of every workout. Now I'm going to show you how easy they are to do and how little time they actually take. Of course, if you have been injured recently or have a medical condition for which stretching, warming up, or working out might not be recommended, be sure to check with your doctor before initiating any of these activities.

Warming Up

Many people think that stretching should come before a warm-up, but the opposite is actually true. Warming up before stretching gets your blood circulating and raises the temperature of your muscles and body, making your muscles more pliable and enabling them to stretch farther.

What constitutes warming up? It can be as simple as doing the activity you plan on doing but at a lighter intensity. If you're going to use a treadmill, get your blood flowing by walking at a slower pace than you'll be walking at during your workout. If you're going to use a rowing machine, row at a pace that, in ten minutes, would enable you to cross a small pond, not the English Channel. Start off slowly and then gradually build your intensity.

There are many different ways to warm-up. Let's say your exercise is a five-mile bicycle ride, which means your warm-up might be a leisurely tour twice around the block. But if you don't want to have to stop and get off your bike after your warm-up to stretch, you can try a different warm-up instead. You could take a slow walk that develops into a jog, or you could do jumping jacks or even a version of your favorite dance step—in short, anything that will keep you moving for about five minutes. That's all the time you need for a good warm-up. Also, try to use the larger muscles in your lower body during your warm-up. You need to get your blood circulating throughout your body, and you need to work the larger muscles to accomplish this effectively.

Finally, for strength training, after you have done your general warm-up, it's a good idea to start each specific exercise using lighter weights before you begin your "official" repetitions. This step is especially important for beginners so they can get accustomed to the motions involved in each exercise.

Stretching

You already know why stretching is important: it gives you better flexibility, thereby increasing your range of motion and decreasing your chances of injury. Stretching improves your posture and promotes good health in general by lengthening the muscles that typically shorten with age. Stretching also targets tight muscles in the lower back that are common causes of lower back pain.

So if stretching is so good for you, why do so many people dislike it? My opinion is that they think stretching is more complicated than it actually is. There are many excellent texts crammed with descriptions of hundreds of healthful stretches, but to the beginner or someone who doesn't have much time (or to the beginner who doesn't have much time), this amount of information can be overwhelming. Since many people follow the all-or-nothing principle, they choose to skip stretches because they figure they could never do all of them.

To repeat, it's better to accomplish *something*—even if that something is limited in scope—than to try to be perfect, end up frustrated, and abandon your program. With this in mind, I'm including eight stretches that you can use as a basic, start-off routine. There are probably forty or fifty other stretches that might be better suited to you individually, and I urge you to find out what they might be. But for now, I want you to know a few basic stretches.

Does my stretching routine take a lot of time? Not at all. You can probably do it in about fifteen minutes. Again, make sure that you consult with your doctor before starting a stretching program if you have been injured recently or have a medical condition for which stretching would not be recommended.

Stretching Guidelines

Let's go over some general guidelines before discussing the basic stretching routine. One of the most important is that you should always do your stretches slowly. If you stretch too quickly, you may injure yourself by tearing some of your muscle fibers.

Pay careful attention to what you are feeling in your muscles as you apply your stretch. What you're aiming for is a feeling of slight tension in the muscle you are stretching. You'll know when you reach this point. Don't become overzealous and push yourself to a point of pain. Stretching is a gradual process, and you will improve your flexibility as you continue doing your stretches.

Once you've reached the point during your stretch where you start to feel slight tension, stop and hold your stretch in this position. Don't bounce—continually stretching a muscle and letting it go, stretching it and letting it go. Steadily hold your stretch in the position you've achieved. Of course, if you start to feel some discomfort while you're holding your stretch, adjust it to a more comfortable position. Stretching does not need to be (and should not be) uncomfortable to be effective. The expression "no pain, no gain" applies neither to stretching nor to your fitness program. Hold your stretch steady so the muscle has enough time to lengthen. You will be able to judge your progress by your increased flexibility as time goes on.

How long should you hold your stretches? Most experts recommend that you hold a stretch anywhere from thirty to sixty seconds. Again, if your stretch is painful or you are unable to hold it for even fifteen seconds, adjust it. Have the confidence to know that if you do your stretching routine each time you work out, your flexibility will improve.

Breathing

It is also important that you pay attention to your breathing as you stretch. Breathing brings more oxygen into your body and helps you relax. Obviously, being relaxed will help you perform your stretches more easily. To help yourself relax, you can visualize your muscles becoming looser as you stretch, play soft music in the background, or even burn scented candles (although people may look at you strangely if you're at the gym).

Cooling Down

Finally, it's important that you cool down after you've completed your workout. You should allow your heart rate, breathing rate, and body temperature to gradually return to normal levels, rather than stop suddenly and leave them elevated. Additionally, because blood flow has been increased to the muscles you've been using during your activity, stopping suddenly can lead to pooling of blood in your extremities. This can create dizziness, nausea, and/or fainting. Just as you gradually increased your intensity as you started your exercise, you need to gradually decrease intensity as your workout comes to an end. Again, five minutes is typically enough for an effective cool-down, but you may take longer if you wish—especially if you've been exercising at higher intensities. As with your warm-up, you may continue doing the same activity and cool down simply by decreasing your intensity.

We're now ready to go over the basic stretching routine. I've provided an illustration of each stretch along with a description of how to perform it properly. Since these are common stretches, you may consult a book on stretching if you want further information. Remember to stretch both your right and left sides. And, of course, if you experience shooting pain, numbness, or other unusual symptoms while performing any of these stretches, it's a good idea to see your doctor.

Stretches

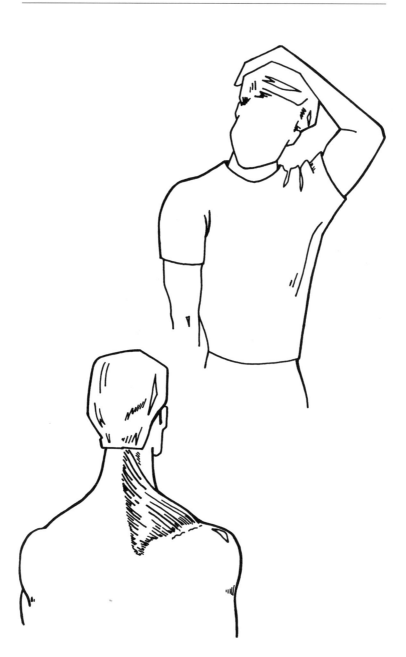

Stretch for Trapezius Muscles

Stretch 1—The Trapezius Muscles

Target

Your trapezius muscles, which extend along the sides of your neck and attach at the top of your shoulders

Significance

These muscles are usually tight because this is where many people carry much of their stress. People who sit a lot or work at a computer tend to have tight trapezius muscles as well.

How to Stretch

Let your head drop toward the shoulder opposite the side you are stretching. If you are stretching your right trapezius muscle, drop your head toward your left shoulder. You can aid the stretch by placing your left hand over the right side of your head or by cupping it over your right ear.

Important Tips

- You can do this stretch standing or seated. If you are doing it standing, bend your knees slightly to take pressure off your lower back. If you are seated, you may hold onto the chair with the hand that's on the same side as the trapezius muscle you're stretching; this will help stretch this muscle even more.
- Be careful not to raise the shoulder that's on the same side as the trapezius muscle you're stretching. The shoulder may go up a bit naturally, but try to focus on relaxing, not tensing, the muscle.
- Keep your head facing forward when you perform this stretch. If your head is rotated, it can place pressure on the sensitive joints in your neck.

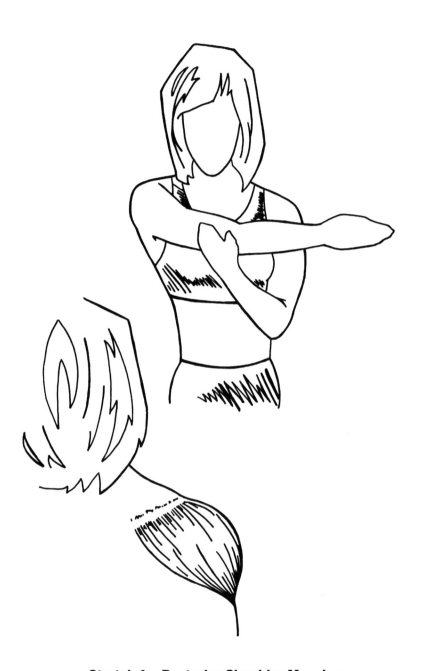

Stretch for Posterior Shoulder Muscles

Stretch 2—The Posterior Shoulder Muscles

Target

The muscles that make up the backs of your shoulders and a portion of your upper back

Significance

These muscles are important for shoulder mobility.

How to Stretch

Extend the arm of the shoulder you are stretching. Then grasp the elbow of your extended arm with your other hand and bring the extended arm across your body.

Important Tips

- Bring the arm across your body *slowly* until you feel slight tension. Don't jerk your arm quickly into position. Make sure your arm is parallel to the ground. Your elbow should not be tilting upward or dipping down.
- You can do this stretch standing or seated. If you are standing, bend your knees slightly to take some pressure off your lower back.
- Don't twist from your hips. Keep your body straight. Keep your neck relaxed.

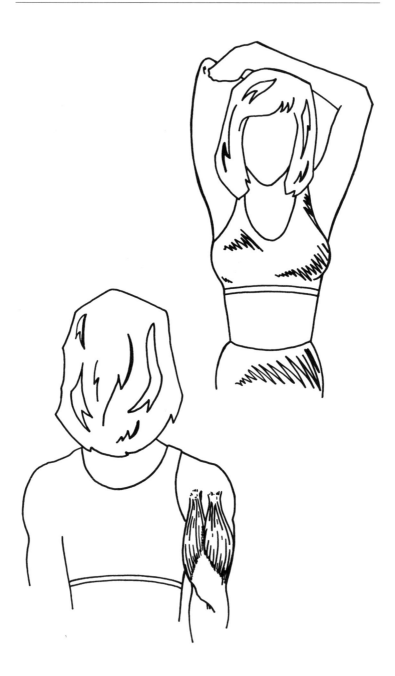

Stretch for Triceps Muscles

Stretch 3—The Triceps Muscles

Target

Your triceps muscles, which are located at the back of your upper arms

Significance

These muscles are important for arm movement.

How to Stretch

Bend the arm you are stretching and bring up the elbow so it is pointing toward the sky and the same-side hand is dangling just below the nape of your neck. Use your other hand to grasp the elbow and pull backward slowly, applying a steady, gentle stretch.

Important Tips

- The goal is to have your elbow pointing upward, but don't force it into this position. Do what you can; eventually, you'll be able to do more.
- Remember to apply a gentle stretch; don't force your elbow back.
- If you are standing, bend your knees slightly to take pressure off your lower back.

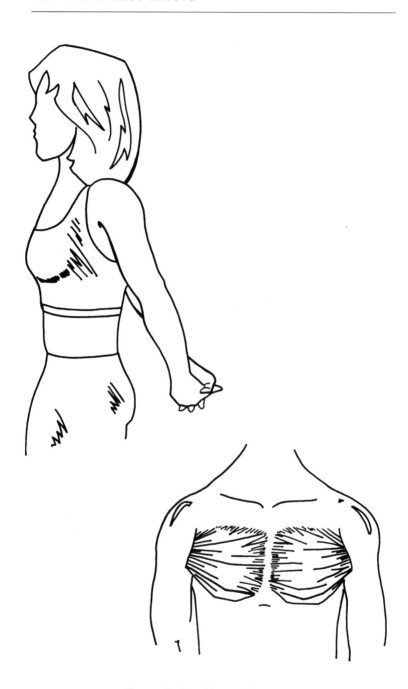

Stretch for Chest Muscles

Stretch 4—The Chest

Target

Your chest and the muscles of your rib cage

Significance

This area is very important for upper body movement. Also, because people sit for extended periods of time, many develop rounded shoulders, putting pressure in the midback area.

How to Stretch

Stand and put your hands behind your back and interlace your fingers. Then slowly extend your arms backward, allowing your chest to protrude.

Important Tips

- Bring your hands back *slowly,* being sure that you never create more than slight tension.
- Don't raise your arms too far upward. This will create a shrugging motion in your shoulders and put pressure on your neck.
- Keep your neck and shoulders relaxed and bend your knees slightly to take pressure off your lower back.
- Notice that as you inhale, you are stretching your rib cage.

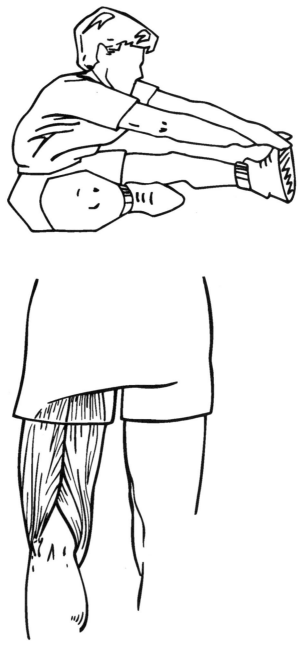

Stretch for Hamstring Muscles

Stretch 5—The Hamstrings

Target

The hamstring muscles, located at the back of your thighs

Significance

Tight hamstrings are a common cause of lower back pain and also limit trunk motion.

How to Stretch

You may effectively stretch the hamstrings either seated or standing. If you are seated, sit on the floor and extend the leg you're stretching while bending your other leg so the foot is resting against the inside of your extended leg's thigh (your leg should be bent at about a ninety-degree angle). Bend forward from the waist as you bring your arms toward the foot of your extended leg.

If you are standing, place your weight on the leg you are not stretching and hold the leg you are stretching at about a thirty-degree angle from the supporting leg. Placing your leg on a carton or a good-sized step will help you achieve the proper angle. Lean down toward your angled leg, allowing your arms to move down the front of your thigh to a point where you feel slight tension in the back of your thigh.

Important Tips

• When sitting, remember to bend forward from your waist, not your neck and shoulders.
• When standing, slightly flex the knee of the supporting leg.
• No matter which position you're using, be careful not to force the stretch so that you're in pain. If you're one of the many people who have tight hamstrings, you can tear muscle fibers if you become overzealous. Also, remember not to bounce with this stretch.

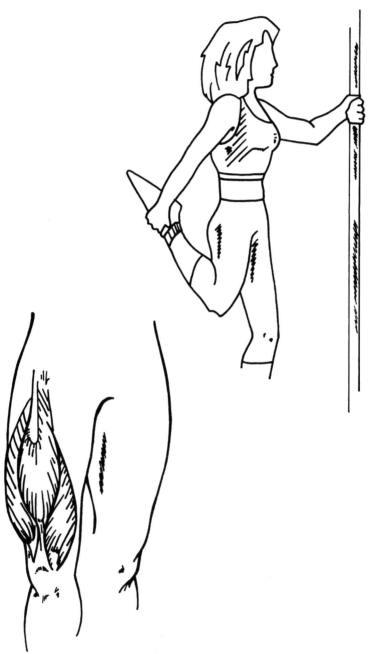

Stretch for Quadriceps Muscles

Stretch 6—The Quadriceps Muscles

Target

The quadriceps muscles, located at the front of your thighs

Significance

Like the hamstrings, the quadriceps are instrumental in moving the lower body. When you're stretching the hamstrings, it's also good to stretch the quadriceps, which work in opposition to them.

How to Stretch

Be sure to stabilize yourself by holding onto something for support before you start this stretch. While standing, bend the knee of the leg you wish to stretch, lift the foot, and bend the foot up and backward toward your buttocks. Grasp the ankle of the leg you're stretching and gently pull it up closer to your buttocks.

Important Tips

- Don't worry if you can't pull your ankle all the way up to your buttocks. As you continue with your stretching program, your flexibility will improve.
- Try to keep your body upright as you perform this stretch; don't tilt too far forward. Bend the knee of your supporting leg a bit to take pressure off your lower back.

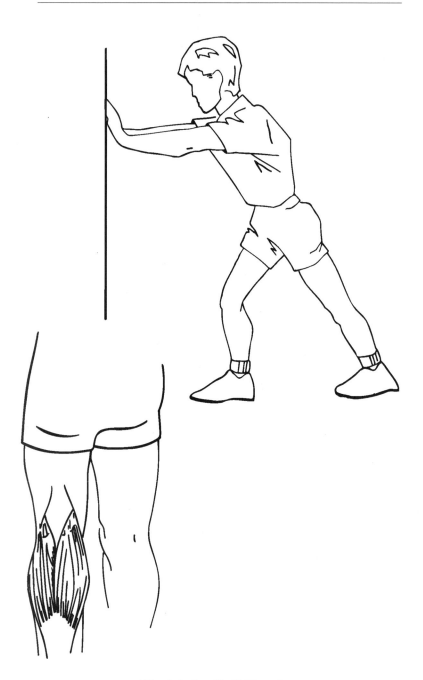

Stretch for Calf Muscles

Stretch 7—The Calf Muscles

Target

Your calf muscles, located at the back of your legs, below your knees

Significance

Tight calves can cause muscular pain and cramping (often referred to as a charley horse). Your calves are also very important for balance.

How to Stretch

This stretch should be done standing. Place your hands flat against a wall or similar support. The leg you're stretching should be extended behind you with the foot flat on the floor. Your supporting leg should be bent and in front of the one you're stretching. Lean gently into the stretch.

Important Tips

- If you don't feel you're getting the stretch you want, try moving the supporting foot forward or the leg that's being stretched farther back. You may also bend your supporting knee more to get a better stretch.
- Point both feet straight ahead.
- Keep your back foot—the foot of the leg you're stretching— flat on the ground. To accomplish this, you may need to move it in a bit toward your supporting leg.

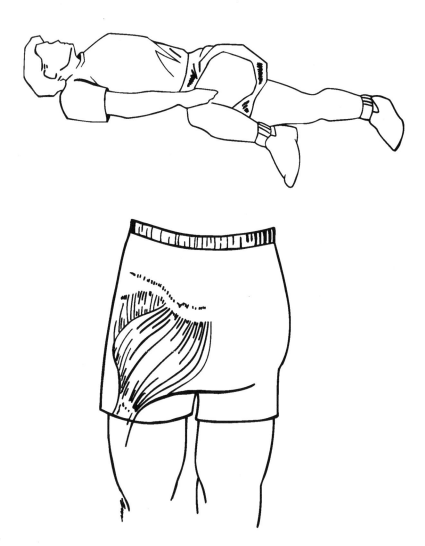

Stretch for Gluteal Muscles

Stretch 8—The Gluteal Muscles

Target

Your gluteal muscles (buttocks) and the muscles around your hips

Significance

When these muscles are tight, they can contribute to lower back pain. They are also involved in leg extension and rotation.

How to Stretch

Lying on your back, bring one knee up and cross it over your extended other leg. Place your opposite-side hand near your knee and press down gently to apply the stretch.

Important Tips

- You may need to raise or lower your knee a bit to isolate the muscle you're stretching.
- Try to keep your upper body relaxed.
- Many people have tightness in the gluteal area and aren't able to stretch as far as they would like to. This is fine; work at your own pace. Don't get discouraged and place too much pressure on or near your knee. You'll be able to stretch farther as you continue with your stretching program.

It's Time to Find Your Fitness Groove

You now have all the tools you need to successfully start, follow through with, and achieve measurable results from your fitness program. If, for some reason, you have still not recorded the SEARCH tapes, please take the time and record them now. Remember, establishing a strong, emotionally appealing reason for sticking with your program and continuously having awareness of this reason is your key for getting into, and staying in, the Fitness Groove.

I commend you on your decision to participate in regular exercise. You'll gain so many benefits—many of which you may not even be aware of—that will dramatically improve the functioning and the quality of your life.

Don't forget that your fitness program doesn't need to be difficult for you to achieve results. If you're able to perform only moderate levels of exercise a few times a week, that's fine. Do what you can and be proud of yourself for exercising and for sticking with your program. You can always increase the levels of your exercise as you continue with your workouts.

I wish you much success in all your endeavors. Please feel free to write me personally with any success stories or comments you may have.

APPENDIX I

SEARCH Technique I: How to Find and Lock In Your Motivation

This is the first script you will record. Before you begin to read aloud, take a few deep breaths, inhaling through your nose and exhaling slowly through your mouth. As you record the script, be aware of the rhythm of your voice and try to read at a leisurely, comfortable pace. If you find yourself rushing, stop recording, rewind the tape, and begin again.

Close your eyes now. And with your eyes closed, perhaps you'll notice how good it feels to have a moment just to sit or lie comfortably and relax. We get so caught up in the rush of daily life and attending to tasks that we forget how to relax and how to pay attention to what is really most important.

Now imagine yourself sitting back in your favorite chair. It could be a chair that you own or one that exists in your imagination. Allow this chair to be the most comfortable, cozy chair you've ever had the pleasure of relaxing in. The soft, smooth fabric cradles and supports your body, helping you feel peaceful and at ease. If the chair has a footrest, maybe you'd like to swing your legs up and rest your feet there. Perhaps you have some small, well-stuffed pillows to support your back and your neck. Whatever it is that allows you to be the most comfortable now, go ahead and enjoy all the wonderful feelings of just being relaxed. Feel that perfect chair supporting the weight of your body as you relax more and more.

Maybe you'll begin to notice a pleasant sensation starting at the tips of your toes. It's a pleasant sensation that spreads into all the areas of your feet, moving across the soles and arches, bathing your feet in comfort and relaxation.

Now allow this sensation to spread into your ankles and your calves, as if your perfect chair has a motor inside that massages each and every muscle it is supporting . . . completely relaxing your ankles and your calves and spreading now into your thighs and buttocks. Feel this wave of relaxation releasing all the muscles of your ankles, your calves, your thighs, and your buttocks, and feel your legs completely at rest.

Now allow this sensation to spread throughout your lower back, move across and around to the front of your body, and spread into the muscles of your abdomen and your stomach, relaxing these areas deeply and thoroughly. Let this wave of relaxation flow into your middle back, bathing every muscle in complete and total comfort as you continue to relax more and more . . . moving now into the muscles of your upper back, across your shoulders, and down into your upper arms, your forearms, your hands, and into the tip of each finger as your hands and your arms fully relax.

Now feel this wave of relaxation spreading across the muscles that join your neck to your shoulders, into your neck, and into all the small muscles of your face as they relax deeply and comfortably. And maybe you can feel the tiny muscles growing more and more deeply relaxed.

Your entire body is now completely and thoroughly relaxed. Every muscle, from the tips of your toes; up through your ankles and your calves; up into your thighs and your buttocks; across your lower back, your middle back, and your upper back; across your shoulders; into your arms and your hands, your neck and your face . . . every part of your body is completely and thoroughly relaxed.

Now, in your mind, travel to a restful place. It can be a real place that you've actually visited, a place that you'd like to visit one day, or a make-believe place that exists only in your imagination. You can wander a beach of ivory sand on one of the Fiji Islands or maybe lie in a cotton hammock that's stretched between two towering oak trees by a secluded mountain cabin.

Or maybe you're at home, curled up on the couch with someone you care about and a book you've been meaning to read since high school. It doesn't matter whether you're someone who loves being out in nature or cocooning indoors by the fire, and it doesn't matter whether you're a person who can visualize easily or a person who prefers to just get a sense of things. Whatever kind of person you are and whatever kind of place makes you feel most relaxed, allow yourself to be there now and experience the peace and comfort that this place provides.

Now that you're in your restful place, look around. If you're outside, what do you see? What color is the sky? Are there any clouds floating there? And if there are, do they appear to arrange themselves into a particular pattern or shape? Look around you and notice all the remarkable aspects of nature. What do you see that interests you? Notice the light. Is the sun shining, or is it sinking toward the horizon, or has night already fallen?

If you're indoors, notice your surroundings. What is the room like? What can you see? Maybe there are items of sentimental value that are special to you or maybe objects of beauty and works of art meant to please the eye and soothe the soul.

Notice the sounds that greet your ears. What do you hear? Are you surrounded by nature and the rustling of wind through leaves and grass? If there are others with you, maybe you can hear the pleasant sound of their voices murmuring in conversation or lilting in laughter. Or maybe you're alone and the only sounds are those of your own breath entering and leaving your body over and over again.

And as you continue to breathe, become aware of the smells that greet you. Are there any special fragrances that you associate with this place? Maybe you can smell a salty gust from the sea or the crisp, piney edge of a mountain breeze.

What else do you perceive? The sand sinking gently beneath your feet . . . your limbs suspended in the soft embrace of a hammock? . . . Whatever you feel, wherever you are, allow yourself to experience the peace and comfort that this place provides.

And allow yourself to be there on the perfect day, at the perfect time of the year, in the perfect setting to make decisions about what matters most to you. We have so many opportunities to make decisions that can lead us toward the lives we really want. Now is your chance to make one of those decisions. Now, right now, commit to the date you have chosen to start your exercise program. Commit to starting your program on *Monday, the first of March,* * and know that you've also made a commitment to living a better life, a life of improved health, vitality, and happiness.

And just as it's important to commit to a starting date, it's also important to know what your personal reasons are for wanting to improve your health and fitness.

---

*Or the seventh of August, or the thirty-first of May. Whatever date you have chosen to start your program, say it here.

We all have reasons for doing what we do, and every once in a while, it's good to remind ourselves of these reasons.

You already know that becoming fit is a good idea if you want to improve your health and physical appearance. You can experience so many exciting benefits that it's worth spending some time exploring all your reasons.

Are there clothes you wish you could be wearing, clothes that would fit your body perfectly and comfortably if you became fit? Do you wish you could walk confidently into a store and ask for your ideal size?

Would you like to try on new clothes and admire the way they look on you? Are there garments you've hung in the back of the closet because they don't fit the way they used to, or they don't fit the way you'd like them to, or you can't even fit into them at all anymore?

How would it feel to be able to wear these clothes? Maybe you can picture yourself with your body at an improved level of health and fitness. How does it feel to have people compliment you on how great you look and say what a difference they can see in your appearance? Do you carry yourself differently now, perhaps with more confidence and a greater sense of purpose?

How are your relationships with your coworkers, now that you've become fit and healthy? Do people look at you differently when you pass them in the hall? How about your relationships with your family and friends? When you go to a party, does your mate introduce you with a touch more pride? Is there someone who treats you a little differently now, perhaps out of respect for what you've accomplished? Could this person even be yourself?

How do you feel when you look in the mirror and see the changes in your appearance? Do you feel proud of yourself and maybe even inspired by your willpower? Do you say to yourself, If I can do this, what else can I accomplish? and go on to achieve other goals that you've always dreamed of but never attempted to reach?

Now that you've become fit and stronger, how healthy do you feel? Can you participate in activities with abundant energy and vitality? Can you gather in deep breaths of air and awaken in the morning feeling refreshed and ready to start the day?

Does your heart feel stronger, and do your lungs feel as if they can accommodate more air? Are you sleeping more deeply and awakening fewer times—or not at all— in the middle of the night? Are you accomplishing more during the day? Are you thinking more clearly, moving more efficiently, and getting the most out of your time?

Isn't it comforting to know that by becoming more fit you've done your body a great service, strengthening and reshaping it, giving yourself the confidence to live an energetic, vital life? . . . Able to enjoy your children and their children for years to come? . . . All from a consistent, manageable investment of energy and time a few times a week.

You now recognize your personal reasons for wanting to become fit and healthy. And maybe you have another, private reason, a reason you haven't mentioned to anyone but one that's important just the same. Whatever your reason may be, it's important that you think of it often. And if you have more than one reason, it's important that you think of them often.

Imagine yourself now fit and healthy. And get a good, clear picture of all the benefits you'll receive as a result of your efforts. And as you create this picture, make the benefits as exciting as your imagination will allow. These benefits that you picture in your mind are your emotionally appealing reasons for maintaining your fitness program.

Now I'd like you to establish a physical signal for yourself that will remind you of these benefits. It could be closing one of your hands into a fist, touching your forehead with your fingertips, or squeezing together your thumb and index finger. It can be whatever you want it to be. Just choose a subtle gesture that you can do almost anywhere at any time. Go ahead and practice it now. Get a clear image of the benefits you'll receive by being fit and healthy, and holding that image in your mind, practice your signal. Do this frequently and you'll develop a strong link between your motivating forces and this simple gesture. Repeat it at night before you fall asleep, in the morning when you awake, and often during the day. It's especially important to use your signal when you listen to this tape. Commit to your signal and it will serve you well.

Anytime you want to feel motivated, use this signal or simply think about your exciting benefits and how good you'll feel when you achieve them. Remember, by keeping your compelling reasons in the front of your mind, you'll always be focused on what's truly important to you and have the motivation you need to stick with your program.

In a moment, you will hear my voice starting to count backward from five to one. As you hear the count, you will turn your awareness outward, back to the external world. And when you hear the count end, you'll open your eyes feeling awake, alert, and fully refreshed.

Five . . . Become aware of your body once again. Are you seated, or are you lying down? In what position are your arms and your legs?

Four . . . What do you hear? Are there sounds nearby, perhaps in the room? Or if you're outdoors, are sounds coming to you from a distance? What is it like to be surrounded by the sound of your own voice?*

Three . . . What do you see behind your closed eyes? Maybe your eyelids are fluttering a bit as they prepare to open.

---

*If someone other than yourself will be recording this script for you, change this sentence to "What is it like to be surrounded by the sound of my voice?"

Two . . . You are aware of listening to an audio cassette. What day is it, and about what time do you think it is?

And, one . . . Open your eyes now, feeling fully awake, alert, and refreshed.

SEARCH Technique II: Designing and Achieving Your Ideal Body

In SEARCH Technique II, I ask you to visualize yourself resting in a hammock. If this is not a relaxing image for you, substitute the opening of SEARCH Technique I, in which you visualize yourself in a comfortable chair.

Go ahead and close your eyes. And with your eyes closed, enjoy the peace of relaxing for a while. During this time, allow yourself to let go and enjoy the feeling of being comfortable and secure.

As you relax, imagine yourself lying safely supported in a spacious hammock that is suspended between two ancient oak trees. These trees are holding the hammock securely as a gentle breeze cools your body. Allow this hammock to be in a place you find relaxing, a place where you are comfortable. Imagine you are there at just the right time, on just the right day, at the perfect time of the year. This is a perfect time to focus on what is most important in your life.

Perhaps you can feel a gentle swaying now as the hammock begins to rock you ever so slightly back and forth . . . suspending you in a feeling of total comfort and relaxation as your entire body is supported safely and comfortably by the cradling hammock.

And maybe you can become aware now of a sensation starting in the tips of your toes . . . a pleasant sensation that spreads across the tops of your feet, around the sides of your feet, and into your soles and heels—a feeling of complete and total relaxation bathing your feet.

Allow this comfort and relaxation to move into your ankles and calves as the hammock rocks you gently. Now allow this sensation to move upward, completely relaxing your ankles and your calves and spreading now into your thighs so both of your legs are completely and thoroughly relaxed. Feel this wave of relaxation releasing all the muscles of your ankles, your calves, and your thighs . . . and moving now into your buttocks as they sink comfortably into the fabric of the hammock, secure and supported as the hammock rocks you gently into a feeling of deeper and deeper relaxation and comfort.

Allow this sensation to spread into your lower back and feel completely at ease as you enjoy being cradled and suspended, as if you're floating on air. Now allow this wave of relaxation to continue up into the middle of your back as it is supported by the hammock, every muscle cradled in security and comfort . . . feel it moving now into the muscles of your upper back, across your shoulders, and down into your upper arms, your elbows, your forearms, and your hands. And allow your arms to lie loosely and comfortably at your sides . . . feeling very comfortable, very peaceful, and very secure.

Now feel this wave of relaxation spreading across the muscles that join your neck to your shoulders, into your neck, and into all the small muscles of your face as they relax deeply and comfortably. And maybe you can feel the tiny muscles growing more and more deeply relaxed.

Your entire body is now completely and thoroughly relaxed. Every muscle, from the tips of your toes; up through your ankles and your calves; up into your thighs and your buttocks; across your lower back, your middle back, and your upper back; across your shoulders; into your arms and your hands, your neck and your face . . . every part of your body is completely and thoroughly relaxed.

In a moment, you'll be traveling to a different place, and you'll hear my voice starting to count from one to five. If you're able to visualize easily, you might like to picture yourself walking down a grassy hill into a beautiful meadow. Or you might like to imagine yourself kneeling on a beach, tracing each number in the sand with your finger, watching the tide flow in and wash away each number as you trace the next. Maybe you won't visualize much of anything at all, and that's fine, too. But still, you'll hear the sound of my voice, and you'll allow yourself to relax more and more.

Now the count will begin . . . and as you hear the count, you will release the tension from your body, starting with your head and working downward toward your feet, relaxing every muscle, letting all the tension go.

One . . . Allow the muscles of your face and neck to relax now, even more than before. Allow the muscles to relax deeply and comfortably. Enjoy this feeling of calm and comfort.

Two . . . Allow the muscles of your shoulders, your arms, your hands, and your fingers to relax now to a much deeper level than before. Relax all these muscles, deeper and deeper, completely and fully.

Three . . . Allow the muscles of your upper back and your middle back to relax even more fully. Let all these muscles release their tension and grow loose as they relax more and more deeply.

Four . . . Now relax your entire lower back and buttocks, releasing all the tension, relaxing more thoroughly with every breath you take.

And, five . . . Now allow your thighs, your calves, your ankles, and your feet to give in to the comfort, releasing all their tension and growing more deeply and thoroughly relaxed. And you might find it interesting to notice that, even though your body is very relaxed, your mind is still active and focused on what's important in your life.

Now picture yourself at your place of comfort. Maybe it's that ivory beach in Fiji, and you're strolling along the shore with the cool, clear water lapping at your feet. Or maybe you're up in the mountains, enveloped in whiteness, with the snow muffling your footsteps as you climb higher and higher into the clean, thin air. Or maybe your place of comfort is your backyard, where you're reclining peacefully in a comfortable lounge chair. Or perhaps you feel happiest curled up on the couch in front of a blazing fire on a snowy winter night. Wherever your place of comfort is, allow yourself to be in this place now, completely relaxed.

And as you relax in your place of comfort, picture a large wooden door before you . . . a door that you walk toward and push with your outstretched hand and that opens into a room where you feel instantly and completely at ease. The room could be one that you've visited before or one that exists only in your imagination.

In the center of this room stands a magnificent three-paneled mirror, similar to the ones that you'd see in a tailor's or a dressmaker's shop. In front of the mirror's central panel is a velvet pedestal. Both the mirror and the pedestal are bathed in soft light.

Now, in your mind, remove your shoes and step onto the pedestal, enjoying the feeling of the plush velvet cradling your feet. Slowly raise your eyes and look into the mirror.

As you see your reflection, perhaps you can observe some of the characteristics of your body's appearance. Notice the shape of your shoulders and your arms, the definition of your chest and your abdomen, the muscle tone in your thighs and your legs, the contours of your hips and your buttocks.

As you gaze at your reflection, accept all the feelings you're having. There may be aspects of your body's appearance that you'd like to change, and that's fine.

Try to look deeper and visualize the intricate inner workings of your body . . . your heart beating, pumping blood to all your tissues and organs . . . your lungs expanding and contracting, in and out, capturing oxygen that will be used for nourishment and energy . . . and, of course, the vast network of arteries and veins guiding your blood around your body.

And by focusing on these marvelous processes you may be able to develop an even greater appreciation of how remarkable your body really is . . . the magnificent way all your cells, muscles, organs, and tissues work together to form your physical body.

Continue gazing in the mirror, and as you do, see if you can look even deeper, down beneath the layers of your skin and muscle and bone, down to the essence of the person you truly are . . . the person who gives and receives love, the person who touches others with a simple gesture or a kind word . . . the person who delights in laughing at a good joke and being a trusted friend. The same person who has made a commitment to taking care of his or her body.

Basically, your body is like a magnificent overcoat that you wear throughout your life. The exciting thing is, if you don't like the shape of the coat, you can alter it. If the coat has extra padding in the waist, you can move the padding up to the shoulders. If the coat is too generously cut, its silhouette can be trimmed. These alterations can be accomplished with an investment of time and energy. Your commitment is all that is needed to redesign the coat into one that will enhance and not hide the person you truly are.

And as you continue looking into the mirror, notice now an elegant golden clothing rack standing next to you. Suspended from this rack is a jewel-encrusted hanger, and on this hanger is draped something you can't quite see because it's hidden by a soft, velvet cover. Reach your hand out toward the rack now and push the velvet cover aside to reveal an article of clothing that has special meaning for you. Maybe it's the dress or the suit you were married in; maybe it's a pair of jeans that used to fit just right a long time ago; or maybe it's a pair of shorts that you feel attractive in. It doesn't have to be something from the past. It can be something that you still wear or something you've kept tucked away because you were waiting for the day when you could finally fit into it again.

Go ahead and put on this article of clothing now and experience how good it feels to have it fit you comfortably and perfectly. Admire the fit in the mirror and see how good you look.

If you want to see this clothing fit even better, change your body however you'd like to—trim it down or build it up, or trim it down in some places and bulk it up in others—so that you really look your best. Make this image an extremely appealing one. And realize, too, that your ideal body is the body that's ideal for *you*. Everybody's different, and everyone has a different body. You don't have to be a high-fashion model or an Olympic gymnast to be in excellent physical shape. Maybe your goal is to lose fifteen pounds or make a few changes to a few areas of your body. That's fine. Maybe you already see your body as ideal for you—and that's fine, too.

Now, let yourself feel how you'd carry yourself if you had the body you desire. How healthy are you? Do you have energy and vitality? Is your heart strong? Do your lungs feel strong? Are you able to easily gather in nourishing breaths of air?

Once you've gotten an exciting, appealing image of yourself and you can imagine how good it would feel to look that way, establish a physical signal that you can use to recall this feeling whenever you'd like to. Perhaps you'd like to close one of your hands into a fist or touch your forehead with your fingertips or squeeze together your thumb and index finger. The signal can be whatever you want it to be. Just choose a subtle gesture that you can do at any time. Go ahead and try it now, reinforcing this appealing image, keeping it at the front of your mind. Any time you wish to be reminded of the physical benefits that you'll reap from your exercise program, use this signal.

Remember, by keeping your focus on your appealing reasons for becoming fit and healthy, you'll be able to follow through with your program. Every time you exercise, keep this picture in the front of your mind. See yourself working toward and accomplishing your goals.

In a moment, you will hear my voice starting to count backward from five to one. As you hear the count, you'll turn your awareness outward, back to the external world. And when you hear the count end, you'll open your eyes feeling awake, alert, and fully refreshed.

Five . . . Become aware of your body once again. Are you seated, or are you lying down? In what position are your arms and your legs?

Four . . . What do you hear? Are there sounds nearby, perhaps in the room? . . . Or if you're outdoors, are sounds coming to you from a distance? What is it like to be surrounded by the sound of your own voice?*

Three . . . What do you see behind your closed eyes? Maybe your eyelids are fluttering a bit as they prepare to open.

Two . . . You are aware of listening to an audio cassette. What day is it, and about what time do you think it is?

And, one . . . Open your eyes now, feeling fully awake, alert, and refreshed.

---

*If someone other than you will be recording this script, change this sentence to "What is it like to be surrounded by the sound of my voice?

APPENDIX II

Using the Personal Success Logbook

Your Personal Success Logbook will help you keep track of your progress, an important part of the follow-through process. You will notice that the logbook is not divided into weekly segments but rather into numbered workouts for either aerobic or strength training sessions. This will encourage you to build flexibility into your workout schedule (see chapter 5).

To use the logbook, choose aerobic or strength training for your first workout. Record your results from this session onto the appropriate page in your logbook, and you'll be ready for your second workout. Don't worry about which kind of workout you should choose (refer to the cross-training instructions in chapter 10) or on which days you should work out. You should be concerned only with the number of workouts you want to do each week.

If you participate in aerobic training and strength training on the same day, use both log sheets to record your results. If you decide your first workout will be strictly aerobic, record your results on the aerobic training sheet for workout number one, and cross out the strength training sheet for workout number one. This way you'll always know how many workouts you've done.

Don't worry about wasting paper; the logbook includes enough sheets to last for three weeks if you're doing four workouts a week or for one month if you're doing three workouts a week. Of course, you can always remove a blank page for aerobic training and a blank page for strength training and make photocopies to extend your logbook.

Let's review how to fill in the log sheets.

Aerobic Training Log Sheet

Date/Activity

The date is self-explanatory. If you're using a stair-stepper for your workout, write "stair-stepper" as your activity.

Level/Setting

Some machines can be operated at different levels or settings. If you are using an elliptical machine at a resistance level of three, write "resistance level 3" in this space so you can refer to it during your next workout.

Duration

This refers to how long you performed your aerobic activity.

Distance/Calories

This pertains to equipment such as treadmills and stair-steppers that can give you readings of the distance you covered as well as the number of calories you burned while you were using the equipment. Write down these readings whenever you use this sort of equipment so you can compare them with the levels you achieve at future workout sessions. When you make your comparisons, be sure to take into consideration how intensely you were exercising on the days when you took the readings.

Intensity

On the log sheets, the numerical scale runs from one through twenty. However, as discussed in chapter 9, you may use a scale of one through ten or fifteen if you'd prefer. It doesn't matter how many numbers you use for your RPE (rating of perceived exertion) as long as your scale makes sense to you.

Notes

Use this section to note any observations or insights you have. If treadmill number three at your gym tends to shut off ten minutes after you start using it, you might want to make a note of it so you don't use this machine again.

Measurements

Record your waist and hip measurements here (as described in chapter 7).

Body Fat Testing

Use this space to record the sites you're using to take skinfold caliper readings as well as the locations of your pinches (for example, three inches down from the top of your shoulder) and your measurements. There is also space to record your body fat percentage based upon your measurements. (Refer to the instructions included with your calipers.)

Pulse Rates

Use this space to record your resting pulse and recovery pulse rates (described in chapter 7).

Strength Training Log Sheet

Date

The date is self-explanatory.

Target

Use this space to record the areas of your body that you're targeting. If you're splitting your routines and working on your lower body this time, you might write "lower body." If you're concentrating on your chest and triceps, you might write "chest and tri's." (Tri's is a slang term for triceps.)

Exercise/Wt/Rep

First, write the type of strength training exercise. Then use the Wt/Rep (weight/repetitions) spaces to record each set. There is room to record four sets for each exercise. (For more than four sets, continue on the next line.) An entry for three sets on the incline bench press might look like this:

Incline bench press 100/9 100/9 100/8

Such an entry would indicate that this person had lifted 100 pounds for nine repetitions in the first set, 100 pounds for nine reps in the second set, and 100 pounds for eight reps in the third set.

Measurements

You can monitor increases in your muscle mass by recording body measurements here. Use the "location" space to identify where you are taking your measurement—for instance, four inches from the top of your shoulder. You can take multiple measurements of the same muscle or muscle group by noting the different locations you are using.

Personal Success Logbook

Aerobic Training 1

Date: _____ *Activity:* _____

LEVEL/SETTING: _____

DURATION: _____ **DISTANCE/CALORIES:** _____

INTENSITY: 1   2   3   4   5   6   7   8   9   10
                11   12   13   14   15   16   17   18   19   20

NOTES: _____

_____

MEASUREMENTS:

WAIST: _____   **HIP:** _____

BODY FAT TESTING:

SITE: _____   **LOCATION:** _____   **MSMT:** _____

SITE: _____   **LOCATION:** _____   **MSMT:** _____

SITE: _____   **LOCATION:** _____   **MSMT:** _____

SITE: _____   **LOCATION:** _____   **MSMT:** _____

SITE: _____   **LOCATION:** _____   **MSMT:** _____

BODY FAT PERCENTAGE: _____

PULSE RATES:

RESTING: _____   **RECOVERY:** _____

Strength Training

Date: *Target:*

EXERCISE	WT/REP	WT/REP	WT/REP	WT/REP
_____	_____	_____	_____	_____
_____	_____	_____	_____	_____
_____	_____	_____	_____	_____
_____	_____	_____	_____	_____
_____	_____	_____	_____	_____
_____	_____	_____	_____	_____
_____	_____	_____	_____	_____
_____	_____	_____	_____	_____
_____	_____	_____	_____	_____
_____	_____	_____	_____	_____
_____	_____	_____	_____	_____
_____	_____	_____	_____	_____
_____	_____	_____	_____	_____
_____	_____	_____	_____	_____

MEASUREMENTS:

MUSCLE	LOCATION	MSMT
_____	_____	_____
_____	_____	_____
_____	_____	_____
_____	_____	_____
_____	_____	_____
_____	_____	_____
_____	_____	_____

Aerobic Training 2

Date: _____ *Activity:* _____

LEVEL/SETTING: _____

DURATION: _____ **DISTANCE/CALORIES:** _____

INTENSITY: 1   2   3   4   5   6   7   8   9   10
              11   12   13   14   15   16   17   18   19   20

NOTES: _____

_____

MEASUREMENTS:

WAIST: _____   **HIP:** _____

BODY FAT TESTING:

SITE: _____   **LOCATION:** _____   **MSMT:** _____

SITE: _____   **LOCATION:** _____   **MSMT:** _____

SITE: _____   **LOCATION:** _____   **MSMT:** _____

SITE: _____   **LOCATION:** _____   **MSMT:** _____

SITE: _____   **LOCATION:** _____   **MSMT:** _____

BODY FAT PERCENTAGE: _____

PULSE RATES:

RESTING: _____   **RECOVERY:** _____

Strength Training

Date: Target:

EXERCISE	WT/REP	WT/REP	WT/REP	WT/REP
_____	_____	_____	_____	_____
_____	_____	_____	_____	_____
_____	_____	_____	_____	_____
_____	_____	_____	_____	_____
_____	_____	_____	_____	_____
_____	_____	_____	_____	_____
_____	_____	_____	_____	_____
_____	_____	_____	_____	_____
_____	_____	_____	_____	_____
_____	_____	_____	_____	_____
_____	_____	_____	_____	_____
_____	_____	_____	_____	_____
_____	_____	_____	_____	_____
_____	_____	_____	_____	_____
_____	_____	_____	_____	_____

MEASUREMENTS:

MUSCLE	LOCATION	MSMT
_____	_____	_____
_____	_____	_____
_____	_____	_____
_____	_____	_____
_____	_____	_____
_____	_____	_____
_____	_____	_____

Aerobic Training

Date: *Activity:*

LEVEL/SETTING: _____

DURATION: _____ **DISTANCE/CALORIES:** _____

INTENSITY: 1   2   3   4   5   6   7   8   9   10
                11   12   13   14   15   16   17   18   19   20

NOTES: _____

_____

MEASUREMENTS:

WAIST: _____   **HIP:** _____

BODY FAT TESTING:

SITE: _____   **LOCATION:** _____   **MSMT:** _____

SITE: _____   **LOCATION:** _____   **MSMT:** _____

SITE: _____   **LOCATION:** _____   **MSMT:** _____

SITE: _____   **LOCATION:** _____   **MSMT:** _____

SITE: _____   **LOCATION:** _____   **MSMT:** _____

BODY FAT PERCENTAGE:_____

PULSE RATES:

RESTING: _____   **RECOVERY:** _____

Strength Training

Date: _____   *Target:* _____

EXERCISE	WT/REP	WT/REP	WT/REP	WT/REP
_____	_____	_____	_____	_____
_____	_____	_____	_____	_____
_____	_____	_____	_____	_____
_____	_____	_____	_____	_____
_____	_____	_____	_____	_____
_____	_____	_____	_____	_____
_____	_____	_____	_____	_____
_____	_____	_____	_____	_____
_____	_____	_____	_____	_____
_____	_____	_____	_____	_____
_____	_____	_____	_____	_____
_____	_____	_____	_____	_____
_____	_____	_____	_____	_____
_____	_____	_____	_____	_____

MEASUREMENTS:

MUSCLE	LOCATION	MSMT
_____	_____	_____
_____	_____	_____
_____	_____	_____
_____	_____	_____
_____	_____	_____
_____	_____	_____
_____	_____	_____

Aerobic Training

Date: *Activity:*

LEVEL/SETTING: _____

DURATION: _____ **DISTANCE/CALORIES:** _____

INTENSITY: 1   2   3   4   5   6   7   8   9   10

11   12   13   14   15   16   17   18   19   20

NOTES: _____

_____

MEASUREMENTS:

WAIST: _____   **HIP:** _____

BODY FAT TESTING:

SITE: _____   **LOCATION:** _____   **MSMT:** _____

SITE: _____   **LOCATION:** _____   **MSMT:** _____

SITE: _____   **LOCATION:** _____   **MSMT:** _____

SITE: _____   **LOCATION:** _____   **MSMT:** _____

SITE: _____   **LOCATION:** _____   **MSMT:** _____

BODY FAT PERCENTAGE: _____

PULSE RATES:

RESTING: _____   **RECOVERY:** _____

Strength Training

Date: *Target:*

EXERCISE	WT/REP	WT/REP	WT/REP	WT/REP

MEASUREMENTS:

MUSCLE	LOCATION	MSMT

Aerobic Training

Date: Activity:

LEVEL/SETTING: _____

DURATION: _____ **DISTANCE/CALORIES:** _____

INTENSITY: 1   2   3   4   5   6   7   8   9   10

            11   12   13   14   15   16   17   18   19   20

NOTES: _____

_____

MEASUREMENTS:

WAIST: _____   **HIP:** _____

BODY FAT TESTING:

SITE: _____   **LOCATION:** _____   **MSMT:** _____

SITE: _____   **LOCATION:** _____   **MSMT:** _____

SITE: _____   **LOCATION:** _____   **MSMT:** _____

SITE: _____   **LOCATION:** _____   **MSMT:** _____

SITE: _____   **LOCATION:** _____   **MSMT:** _____

BODY FAT PERCENTAGE:_____

PULSE RATES:

RESTING: _____   **RECOVERY:** _____

Strength Training

Date: *Target:*

EXERCISE	WT/REP	WT/REP	WT/REP	WT/REP
_____	_____	_____	_____	_____
_____	_____	_____	_____	_____
_____	_____	_____	_____	_____
_____	_____	_____	_____	_____
_____	_____	_____	_____	_____
_____	_____	_____	_____	_____
_____	_____	_____	_____	_____
_____	_____	_____	_____	_____
_____	_____	_____	_____	_____
_____	_____	_____	_____	_____
_____	_____	_____	_____	_____
_____	_____	_____	_____	_____
_____	_____	_____	_____	_____

MEASUREMENTS:

MUSCLE	LOCATION	MSMT
_____	_____	____
_____	_____	____
_____	_____	____
_____	_____	____
_____	_____	____
_____	_____	____
_____	_____	____

Aerobic Training

Date: *Activity:*

LEVEL/SETTING: _____

DURATION: _____ **DISTANCE/CALORIES:** _____

INTENSITY: 1   2   3   4   5   6   7   8   9   10

11   12   13   14   15   16   17   18   19   20

NOTES: _____

_____

MEASUREMENTS:

WAIST: _____   **HIP:** _____

BODY FAT TESTING:

SITE: _____   **LOCATION:** _____   **MSMT:** _____

SITE: _____   **LOCATION:** _____   **MSMT:** _____

SITE: _____   **LOCATION:** _____   **MSMT:** _____

SITE: _____   **LOCATION:** _____   **MSMT:** _____

SITE: _____   **LOCATION:** _____   **MSMT:** _____

BODY FAT PERCENTAGE: _____

PULSE RATES:

RESTING: _____   **RECOVERY:** _____

Strength Training

Date: _____   *Target:* _____

EXERCISE	WT/REP	WT/REP	WT/REP	WT/REP
_____	_____	_____	_____	_____
_____	_____	_____	_____	_____
_____	_____	_____	_____	_____
_____	_____	_____	_____	_____
_____	_____	_____	_____	_____
_____	_____	_____	_____	_____
_____	_____	_____	_____	_____
_____	_____	_____	_____	_____
_____	_____	_____	_____	_____
_____	_____	_____	_____	_____
_____	_____	_____	_____	_____
_____	_____	_____	_____	_____
_____	_____	_____	_____	_____
_____	_____	_____	_____	_____
_____	_____	_____	_____	_____

MEASUREMENTS:

MUSCLE	LOCATION	MSMT
_____	_____	_____
_____	_____	_____
_____	_____	_____
_____	_____	_____
_____	_____	_____
_____	_____	_____
_____	_____	_____

Aerobic Training

Date: Activity:

LEVEL/SETTING: _____

DURATION: _____ **DISTANCE/CALORIES:** _____

INTENSITY: 1   2   3   4   5   6   7   8   9   10

                  11 12 13 14 15 16 17 18 19 20

NOTES: _____

_____

MEASUREMENTS:

WAIST: _____   **HIP:** _____

BODY FAT TESTING:

SITE: _____   **LOCATION:** _____   **MSMT:** _____

SITE: _____   **LOCATION:** _____   **MSMT:** _____

SITE: _____   **LOCATION:** _____   **MSMT:** _____

SITE: _____   **LOCATION:** _____   **MSMT:** _____

SITE: _____   **LOCATION:** _____   **MSMT:** _____

BODY FAT PERCENTAGE: _____

PULSE RATES:

RESTING: _____   **RECOVERY:** _____

Strength Training

Date: *Target:*

EXERCISE	WT/REP	WT/REP	WT/REP	WT/REP

MEASUREMENTS:

MUSCLE	LOCATION	MSMT

Aerobic Training

8

Date: *Activity:*

LEVEL/SETTING: _____

DURATION: _____ **DISTANCE/CALORIES:** _____

INTENSITY: 1   2   3   4   5   6   7   8   9   10
                11   12   13   14   15   16   17   18   19   20

NOTES: _____

_____

MEASUREMENTS:

WAIST: _____   **HIP:** _____

BODY FAT TESTING:

SITE: _____   **LOCATION:** _____   **MSMT:** _____

SITE: _____   **LOCATION:** _____   **MSMT:** _____

SITE: _____   **LOCATION:** _____   **MSMT:** _____

SITE: _____   **LOCATION:** _____   **MSMT:** _____

SITE: _____   **LOCATION:** _____   **MSMT:** _____

BODY FAT PERCENTAGE: _____

PULSE RATES:

RESTING: _____   **RECOVERY:** _____

Strength Training

Date: _____   *Target:* _____

EXERCISE	WT/REP	WT/REP	WT/REP	WT/REP
_____	_____	_____	_____	_____
_____	_____	_____	_____	_____
_____	_____	_____	_____	_____
_____	_____	_____	_____	_____
_____	_____	_____	_____	_____
_____	_____	_____	_____	_____
_____	_____	_____	_____	_____
_____	_____	_____	_____	_____
_____	_____	_____	_____	_____
_____	_____	_____	_____	_____
_____	_____	_____	_____	_____
_____	_____	_____	_____	_____
_____	_____	_____	_____	_____
_____	_____	_____	_____	_____

MEASUREMENTS:

MUSCLE	LOCATION	MSMT
_____	_____	_____
_____	_____	_____
_____	_____	_____
_____	_____	_____
_____	_____	_____
_____	_____	_____
_____	_____	_____

Aerobic Training

Date: *Activity:*

LEVEL/SETTING: _____

DURATION: _____ **DISTANCE/CALORIES:** _____

INTENSITY: 1   2   3   4   5   6   7   8   9   10

               11   12   13   14   15   16   17   18   19   20

NOTES: _____

_____

MEASUREMENTS:

WAIST: _____   **HIP:** _____

BODY FAT TESTING:

SITE: _____   **LOCATION:** _____   **MSMT:** _____

SITE: _____   **LOCATION:** _____   **MSMT:** _____

SITE: _____   **LOCATION:** _____   **MSMT:** _____

SITE: _____   **LOCATION:** _____   **MSMT:** _____

SITE: _____   **LOCATION:** _____   **MSMT:** _____

BODY FAT PERCENTAGE: _____

PULSE RATES:

RESTING: _____   **RECOVERY:** _____

Strength Training

Date: *Target:*

EXERCISE	WT/REP	WT/REP	WT/REP	WT/REP
_____	_____	_____	_____	_____
_____	_____	_____	_____	_____
_____	_____	_____	_____	_____
_____	_____	_____	_____	_____
_____	_____	_____	_____	_____
_____	_____	_____	_____	_____
_____	_____	_____	_____	_____
_____	_____	_____	_____	_____
_____	_____	_____	_____	_____
_____	_____	_____	_____	_____
_____	_____	_____	_____	_____
_____	_____	_____	_____	_____
_____	_____	_____	_____	_____
_____	_____	_____	_____	_____

MEASUREMENTS:

MUSCLE	LOCATION	MSMT
_____	_____	_____
_____	_____	_____
_____	_____	_____
_____	_____	_____
_____	_____	_____
_____	_____	_____
_____	_____	_____

Aerobic Training

Date: Activity:

LEVEL/SETTING: _____

DURATION: _____ **DISTANCE/CALORIES:** _____

INTENSITY: 1   2   3   4   5   6   7   8   9   10

              11   12   13   14   15   16   17   18   19   20

NOTES: _____

_____

MEASUREMENTS:

WAIST: _____   **HIP:** _____

BODY FAT TESTING:

SITE: _____   **LOCATION:** _____   **MSMT:** _____

SITE: _____   **LOCATION:** _____   **MSMT:** _____

SITE: _____   **LOCATION:** _____   **MSMT:** _____

SITE: _____   **LOCATION:** _____   **MSMT:** _____

SITE: _____   **LOCATION:** _____   **MSMT:** _____

BODY FAT PERCENTAGE: _____

PULSE RATES:

RESTING: _____   **RECOVERY:** _____

Strength Training

Date: Target:

EXERCISE	WT/REP	WT/REP	WT/REP	WT/REP

MEASUREMENTS:

MUSCLE	LOCATION	MSMT

Aerobic Training

Date: *Activity:*

LEVEL/SETTING: _____

DURATION: _____ **DISTANCE/CALORIES:** _____

INTENSITY: 1   2   3   4   5   6   7   8   9   10

            11   12   13   14   15   16   17   18   19   20

NOTES: _____

_____

MEASUREMENTS:

WAIST: _____   **HIP:** _____

BODY FAT TESTING:

SITE: _____   **LOCATION:** _____   **MSMT:** _____

SITE: _____   **LOCATION:** _____   **MSMT:** _____

SITE: _____   **LOCATION:** _____   **MSMT:** _____

SITE: _____   **LOCATION:** _____   **MSMT:** _____

SITE: _____   **LOCATION:** _____   **MSMT:** _____

BODY FAT PERCENTAGE:_____

PULSE RATES:

RESTING: _____   **RECOVERY:** _____

Strength Training

Date: *Target:*

EXERCISE	WT/REP	WT/REP	WT/REP	WT/REP

MEASUREMENTS:

MUSCLE	LOCATION	MSMT

Aerobic Training

Date: Activity:

LEVEL/SETTING: _____

DURATION: _____ **DISTANCE/CALORIES:** _____

INTENSITY: 1   2   3   4   5   6   7   8   9   10
             11   12   13   14   15   16   17   18   19   20

NOTES: _____

_____

MEASUREMENTS:

WAIST: _____   **HIP:** _____

BODY FAT TESTING:

SITE: _____   **LOCATION:** _____   **MSMT:** _____

SITE: _____   **LOCATION:** _____   **MSMT:** _____

SITE: _____   **LOCATION:** _____   **MSMT:** _____

SITE: _____   **LOCATION:** _____   **MSMT:** _____

SITE: _____   **LOCATION:** _____   **MSMT:** _____

BODY FAT PERCENTAGE: _____

PULSE RATES:

RESTING: _____   **RECOVERY:** _____

Strength Training

Date: *Target:*

EXERCISE	WT/REP	WT/REP	WT/REP	WT/REP
_____	_____	_____	_____	_____
_____	_____	_____	_____	_____
_____	_____	_____	_____	_____
_____	_____	_____	_____	_____
_____	_____	_____	_____	_____
_____	_____	_____	_____	_____
_____	_____	_____	_____	_____
_____	_____	_____	_____	_____
_____	_____	_____	_____	_____
_____	_____	_____	_____	_____
_____	_____	_____	_____	_____
_____	_____	_____	_____	_____
_____	_____	_____	_____	_____
_____	_____	_____	_____	_____

MEASUREMENTS:

MUSCLE	LOCATION	MSMT
_____	_____	_____
_____	_____	_____
_____	_____	_____
_____	_____	_____
_____	_____	_____
_____	_____	_____
_____	_____	_____

About the Author

Dr. Scott Lewis is a chiropractic physician whose audiotape version of this program has sold more than 150,000 copies worldwide. He has been in practice for more than eleven years, coached hundreds of people, given seminars around the country, and hosted his own motivational radio show. He has helped Olympic athletes, celebrities, professional athletes, and even Las Vegas showgirls.

Dr. Lewis welcomes your comments and would love to hear from you about your successes.

Lectures, Seminars, Corporate Consultations, Professional Programs

Dr. Lewis is available to present a variety of programs ranging from keynote addresses, lectures, and workshops to in-depth consulting. Each presentation is tailored to the specific needs of the group, whether it's a corporation, a professional association, or the general public.

To contact Dr. Lewis:

Dr. Scott Lewis
2810 W. Charleston Blvd., #H-84
Las Vegas, NV 89102

Phone: 702-456-1200
Fax: 702-877-8815
E-mail: drlewis@drscottlewis.com
Or visit our web site at:
http://www.drscottlewis.com

If you would like more information about Dr. Lewis's seminar schedule, consulting services, and newly released products, please see the order form on the following page.

Order Form for Dr. Lewis's SEARCH™ Tapes

	Qty		Price
How to Find and Lock In Your Motivation (SEARCH I)	____	@ $12.97 =	_____
Designing and Achieving Your Ideal Body (SEARCH II)	____	@ $12.97 =	_____
Two-tape special (Save $2.99)	____	@ $22.95 =	_____

Other bestselling audio programs by Dr. Lewis:

	Qty		Price
Secrets & Techniques for Losing Weight Successfully (2 tapes)	____	@ $24.95 =	_____
The Fitness Follow-Through Formula to Drop Dress Sizes & Pant Sizes (2 tapes)	____	@ $24.95 =	_____
Both programs ($49.90 value - Save $14)	____	@ $35.90 =	_____
Additional copies of this book	____	@ $12.95 =	_____
Shipping/handling (Priority Mail)			3.50
Nevada residents add 7% sales tax			_____
Total enclosed			_____

Make checks/money orders payable to "Breakthrough Enterprises." If using a credit card, please fill out below.

☐ Amex   ☐ Visa   ☐ MasterCard   ☐ Discover

_____   _____
Account No.   Exp. Date

_____
Signature

_____
Name

_____
Address

_____
City, State, Zip

Send your payment with the order form above to
    Breakthrough Enterprises
    2810 W. Charleston Blvd., #H-84
    Las Vegas, NV 89102

If you are using a credit card, for fastest service, fax this form to 702-877-8815.

All orders must be paid in U.S. funds. Please allow 2–3 weeks for delivery.

☐ Send me a free information packet on Dr. Lewis's other products & services and a *surprise gift* too. For FLASH updates, my e-mail address is: _____

Visit our website at www.drscottlewis.com for more information on any of the above audio programs.